ABOUT THE A

Maryon Stewart studied preventive dentistry [...] Hospital in London and worked as a counsell[...] for four years. At the beginning of 1984 sh[...] which has subsequently provided help to thousands of women all over the world. In 1987 she launched the Women's Nutritional Advisory Service, which now provides broader help to women.

As well as writing *Beat PMT Through Diet*, which has been a best-seller since 1987, Maryon has written other popular books including *Beat Sugar Craving*, *Beat IBS Through Diet*, and is the co-author of *The Vitality Diet*, and *The PMT Cookbook*. She has had her own weekly radio programme on Health and Nutrition, has co-written several medical papers and has written articles for many glossy magazines and newspapers including *Marie Clare*, *Cosmopolitan*, *Chat*, *Women's Journal*, *Health & Fitness* and the *Daily Mirror*. She has also appeared on several popular TV magazine shows, including *TV AM*, *GMTV Top of the Morning*, *Good Morning with Anne & Nick*, *Reportage*, *Meridian*, *Carlton*, *BSkyB*, *The Miriam Stoppard Health & Beauty Show*, *This Morning*, *Pebble Mill*, *Channel Four Streetwise*, *TVS*, and in a series of Yorkshire TV's *Help Yourself* programmes.

Maryon now has her own monthly page in the magazine *House and Garden*, and regularly appears on *Capital Woman*. She also lectures to both the lay public and the medical profession. She is married to Dr Alan Stewart, and they live in Lewes, S[...], with their four children.

[...] Stewart qualified as a doctor at Guy's Hospital, London, in 1976, and spent [...] specializing in hospital medicine. He became a member of the Royal College of Physicians (MRCP UK), then worked at the British Homoepathic Hospital in London and qualified as an MF Hom (Member of the Faculty of Homoeopathy). For the last twelve years he has specialized in nutritional medicine and is a founding member of the British Society for Nutritional Medicine. He is also Medical Advisor to The Women's Nutritional Advisory Service and is actively involved in educating other doctors on the subject of nutrition. Dr Stewart co-wrote the best-selling books *Nutritional Medicine* and *The Vitality Diet*, is the author of the book *Tired All the Time*, and has contributed to other books including *Beat Sugar Craving*, *Inside Science*, *The Migraine Revolution* and the academic book *Post Viral Fatigue Syndrome*. He has written several medical papers and regularly gives lectures to doctors and health visitors. Additionally, he has written articles in both the medical and popular press on various aspects of health. He has contributed to many radio programmes, including the BBC *Today* programme, and has also appeared on many TV magazine shows, documentaries, including BBC2's *Healing Arts*, and has taken part in many health debates. He is also a keen organic gardener and an excellent cook.

Guy E. Abraham, MD, is a former Professor of Obstetrics and Gynaecological Endocrinology at UCLA School of Medicine. Because of his research over the past 18 years on the development of sophisticated techniques to measure minute quantities of hormones in blood, he has received worldwide recognition: the General Diagnostic Award of the Canadian Association of Clinical Chemists in 1974; the Medaille d'Honneur of the University of Liège, Belgium, 1976; the Senior Investigator Award of the Clinical Radioassay Society in 1980. The application of these techniques to various female disorders have improved markedly the understanding of these disorders and their management. He is the Patron of the Women's Nutritional Advisory Service.

'No illness which can be treated by diet should be treated by any other means.'
Maimonides, twelfth-century physician

BEAT PMS
THROUGH DIET

The medically proven Women's
Nutritional Advisory Service Programme

Maryon Stewart

with contributions from

Dr Alan Stewart and Dr Guy Abraham

V

VERMILION
LONDON

To daughters everywhere

IMPORTANT NOTE FOR SUFFERERS

There are many fairly technical terms used to describe the Pre-Menstrual Syndrome and the normal menstrual cycle. You may already be familiar with some of the more technical terms, whilst others will be new to you. I have prepared a brief Dictionary of Terms to refer to which begins on page 246. Please don't be afraid to use it as often as necessary. The better you understand the information, the more you will be able to apply it to your own life and symptoms.

If your symptoms occur at other times of the month, apart from during your pre-menstrual time, you should have a medical check-up with your own doctor. If your symptoms are very severe it would be advisable to have your nutritional programme supervised by your own doctor or a trained counsellor. If you get confused or need extra advice, the Women's Nutritional Advisory Service is there to help you. All letters receive a personal reply: their address is on page 254.

This revised edition first published in 1994

1 3 5 7 9 10 8 6 4 2

Text copyright © 1987, 1990 and 1994 by Maryon Stewart, Dr Guy Abraham

The moral right of Maryon Stewart has been asserted in accordance with the Copyright, Designs and Patents Act, 1988.

First published in the United Kingdom in 1987 by Century Publishing Co. Ltd

This edition published in 1994 by Vermilion
an imprint of Ebury Press
Random House, 20 Vauxhall Bridge Road, London SW1V 2SA

Random House Australia (Pty) Limited
10 Alfred Street, Milsons Point, Sydney
New South Wales 2061, Australia

Random House New Zealand Limited
18 Poland Road, Glenfield
Auckland 10, New Zealand

Random House South Africa (Pty) Limited
PO Box 337, Bergvlei, South Africa

Random House UK Limited Reg. No. 954009

A CIP catalogue record for this book
is available from the British Library

ISBN 0 09 178352 6

Illustrations by Mike Gordon

Typeset by SX Composing, Rayleigh, Essex

Printed and bound in Great Britain by Mackays of Chatham plc, Chatham, Kent

CONTENTS

ACKNOWLEDGEMENTS

I would first like to acknowledge the researchers that have gone before us who collectively completed the groundwork that allowed us to begin our work from an advanced point. In particular I refer to early work by Dr Katharina Dalton, Dr Michael Brush, Dr David Horrobin, Dr Guy Abraham and Professor Shaughn O'Brien.

Special thanks are due to both Dr Alan Stewart and Dr Guy Abraham for their advice and support over the years. Without their technical support we would not have been able to provide such valuable help to so many women, and education on the nutritional approach to Pre-Menstrual Syndrome to so many doctors, nurses and medical organizations.

My heartfelt thanks also go to all the wonderful patients who have volunteered to share their case histories with us in this book. Their willingness to divulge intimate details so frankly in an effort to help others is highly appreciated.

Next I must thank the caring team that have worked at the Women's Nutritional Advisory Service, in particular Michele Apsey and Sarah Tooley. Without them this book would not have been possible.

I would also like to thank the following people for advice: Deryn Bell on osteopathy, Paul Lundberg on acupuncture and acupressure and Julia Swift on exercise.

Thanks are also due to Lavinia Trevor for her support and the benefit of her wisdom and to Rowena Webb and Anabel Briggs at Vermilion for their enthusiasm and professionalism.

Lastly, I must thank our wonderful nanny, Joanna John, for happily occupying the children whilst I put the third edition of this book together, and the children themselves, Phoebe, Chesney, Hester and Simeon, for unselfishly allowing me time out, and providing me with regular refreshments and cuddles.

Maryon Stewart

FOREWORD
BY
LESLIE KENTON

This is an extraordinary book. Not only does it tackle the very complex subject of Pre-Menstrual Syndrome (PMS) in a simple and straightforward way so that it becomes understandable to the average woman suffering from it, but it is also eminently practical. It tells you exactly how to go about finding the answer to your own difficulties.

PMS, with its symptoms of bloating, depression, irritability, fatigue and all the rest is not something 'normal' which you have to suffer from, month in month out. I have seen even the most resistant cases turn around through changes of diet, alterations in living habits and the judicious use of certain nutritional supplements. What Maryon Stewart has done so cleverly is to explain how to help yourself: first by making you aware of what your specific problems are, and then by helping you outline a self-directed lifestyle programme for solving them.

And Maryon Stewart can substantiate her claims too. Having already put into practice the natural approach to PMS set out in this book for 11 years, and having monitored its results on a thousand women through the Women's Nutritional Advisory Service, she knows what she is talking about. The methods work. And her advice about eating natural organically-grown foods, using simple techniques which can help you better manage stress, calling on well-planned nutritional supplements when necessary and even making use of natural treatments which you can carry out yourself to cope with acute problems is not only sound in relation to eliminating PMS. It can also be taken far beyond to form the basis of a total lifestyle for optimum health for women and men alike. *Beat PMS Through Diet* is a book to be read, used and then loaned to friends when they need it.

" Judith's Story* "

'After the birth of our first baby I began to experience intense mood swings. One moment I'd be rational and calm, then the next minute I would fly off the handle. My foul mood was lasting two weeks every month. During this time I'd feel bloated and constantly tired. I experienced the most incredible bouts of anger: I'd throw things – there was hardly a decent piece of china left in the house. I'd hit out at everything. All our kitchen equipment was dented and scratched.

I'd rant at my husband and the children. I never hit them, though once I remember raving at my husband with the bread knife in my hand and, at that moment, I could have killed him. Something wouldn't let me, thank God. Sometimes I'd get in the car and fly off down the road. I was lucky I never killed myself or anyone else. I usually clicked back to normal the moment my period started.

My GP suggested my problem was depression, but I knew it wasn't. Luckily for me, by chance I saw a copy of Beat PMS Through Diet in our local bookshop, bought it, read it and phoned up the Advisory Service to get some extra help. That was three years ago. I started on the new regime the next day, and felt better at once. My next period came and went with almost no ill effects. It was magical. The next time I suffered hardly at all. I couldn't believe that after 13 years I was back in the normal world! Both my husband and I agree that our marriage couldn't have lasted much longer if I'd gone on the way I was. I'm just thankful I found out what my problem was before I drove my family away.'

---

* Despite the fact that most of the patients who volunteered to tell their story in the book didn't object to my using their actual names, I felt it would be more appropriate to change their names and let them remain anonymous.

INTRODUCTION

The Pre-Menstrual Syndrome, or PMS, does not have the physical characteristics of an abscess or an ingrown toenail. Neither does it show up under a microscope like a diseased cell. The agony and the anguish suffered, not to mention the misery and the mental torture, cannot easily be measured.

Perhaps because PMS is relatively difficult to detect or quantify by an outsider the condition has taken far longer than it should have done to become recognized, and still longer to be treated effectively without the use of drugs. As a result, women have had to go on suffering unnecessarily.

> 'My doctor told me it was all in my mind. But I gain five inches (12cm) pre-menstrually around the middle. I told him indignantly that if it was anywhere it was all in the waist!'

> 'My monthly symptoms were diagnosed as "problems with my nerves". I was prescribed tranquillizers which I became too dependent upon.'

> 'I was told by my doctor that the solution to my symptoms is to have a baby. I'm single, I don't have a regular boyfriend, and I don't want a baby!'

> 'All part of being a woman' is a hot favourite, followed by 'PMS symptoms are a sign of a woman rejecting her femininity'.

The most inventive advice for overcoming PMS symptoms was the treatment prescribed by a doctor who advised his patient to join the Conservative Party and become a magistrate, as his wife had done previously!

To a non-sufferer this may sound amusing. However, to a woman with

PMS who is feeling wretched, in some cases suicidal, and certainly bitter that her life is being disrupted by this condition, it is really no laughing matter.

There exists now a wealth of evidence to show that PMS not only exists, but that it can be treated, to a large degree, quite naturally. From studies we have undertaken, for example, we have shown that in excess of 90 per cent of the PMS sufferers who follow our recommendations are significantly better within the first three months. The reasons why this approach is not widely recognized are that medical research on PMS has hitherto been scattered far and wide in medical journals around the world, and the medical profession are by their own admission not educated about nutrition; more of this later. By gathering this information together we were able to formulate a very simple, effective programme to help overcome Pre-Menstrual Syndrome.

In order to make this often life-saving information available to anyone and everyone in need, the Women's Nutritional Advisory Service was set up as an interim measure. For 11 years we have been helping thousands of women, not only in Britain, but indeed all over the world.

The Women's Nutritional Advisory Service has carried out a scientific survey of the symptoms, progress and treatment of 1000 women who have consulted them. Throughout the book you will find figures and charts which refer to this survey, unless stated otherwise, as for example, when particular studies were made of individual cases and groups.

We have also been able to provide a Medical Information Service which regularly supplies doctors and other health-care professionals with information about the nutritional approach to PMS. The ideal situation is that the nutritional approach to PMS becomes recognized as a valid part of orthodox medicine and is practised widely.

In the meantime, this book has been put together based on a very successful programme which the Women's Nutritional Advisory Service has been using for the last 11 years. I have hard facts to substantiate our claims, as you will see as you read on. The good news is that overcoming PMS consists mainly of SELF-HELP with a little education along the way.

The book will explain to you how you can solve the problem for yourself, according to your own individual symptoms. It is written in four parts. Part One deals with the realities of Pre-Menstrual Syndrome and the effect it has on individual and family life. Part Two covers nutrition in relation to our body. Part Three is devoted to diet and other means of self-help, and finally, in Part Four, you will find lists of useful information and addresses.

Consider your voyage through this book an adventure, and as we often say to the sufferers beginning our programme – 'May you never be the same again!' Good luck!

1

A PROBLEM
AS OLD AS
THE HILLS

Despite the fact that for the last few years we have been talking and writing about the Pre-Menstrual Syndrome (PMS) as if it has just been discovered, in reality it has been affecting women all over the world for many years.

I am often asked the question 'How come PMS is more common now than it was years ago?' My answer is that we talk about the condition far more now than we used to, and that there are many aspects relating to the twentieth-century diet and environment that seem to contribute significantly to the problem.

The whole event has become affectionately nicknamed 'The Curse'. It seems that this term derives from ancient times when a menstruating woman was considered by society to be unclean, and in some cases dangerous. In some primitive tribes menstrual blood was considered to be evil, and a menstruating woman had to remain shut away for fear that she would cast a spell on the menfolk or kill off whole herds of animals using her temporary 'witch's' powers. If a menstruating woman disobeyed this or similar rules and mixed with the menfolk, some tribes would even condemn her to death.

Certain religions still regard a menstruating woman as undesirable. In the Moslem religion a menstruating woman is not allowed to enter the mosque. As recently as the beginning of this century a Greek Orthodox woman was not permitted Communion during her period, and to this day in the Orthodox Jewish religion, menstruating women are not permitted to sleep with their husbands during their period.

Is it any wonder that complexes about the whole subject developed and that the subject became taboo? Who, with any degree of sanity, would have wanted to admit the fact that their period was due? It makes the mind boggle!

Despite the fact that women's often frenzied accounts of their unbearable pre-menstrual symptoms have been labelled as being 'all in the mind', i.e. a mental condition, past treatments included hysterectomies, electric shock treatment, and even, in tragic cases, lobotomies (an operation where part of the brain is removed). Traditionally Western medicine tends to regard a physical condition as one that we have no control over and that needs treatment by physical means using drugs and suchlike, and a mental condition as one where the person's personality contributes to the illness. This division is seen as being increasingly artificial.

The first recorded cases of PMS (or PMT, as it was then known) were in 1931, when Dr Robert T. Frank, an American physician working in New York reported 15 cases of Pre-Menstrual Tension. These women had symptoms of nervous tension, water retention and weight gain. Dr Frank found a high level of the hormone oestrogen present in these patients and felt that they were unable to excrete the oestrogen from their bodies pre-menstrually. The excess oestrogen, he felt, then irritated the nervous system, and thus symptoms developed.

Further work was done by other American doctors in this field. In 1938 Dr Israel, another American doctor, presented his theory that not all women had high levels of oestrogen, but they did have low levels of the hormone progesterone.

In 1943 Dr Biskind published a study which supported the theory that many pre-menstrual symptoms reported were similar to vitamin B deficiency symptoms. He found that treatment with vitamin B greatly improved symptoms, especially uncomfortable breast symptoms and heavy bleeding during menstruation, which are also symptoms of vitamin B deficiency. The cause was an overload of oestrogen pre-menstrually.

As early as 1944 Dr Harris observed women with pre-menstrual fatigue, nervousness and cravings for sweet foods. Further research along these lines continued in the 1950s.

The first scientific publication from the United Kingdom was in 1937 from a group of women doctors led by Dr McCance from King's College Hospital in London. Their detailed survey of 169 mainly professional women documented the presence of increased fatigue, headaches and mood swings occurring pre-menstrually and during the period. These doctors were uncertain as to the exact cause of these physical and mood changes. In 1953 Dr Katharina Dalton, a British doctor, began publishing her work. She and Dr Raymond Greene renamed the condition 'Pre-Menstrual Syndrome', as they identified so many symptoms as being pre-menstrual. Dr Dalton is considered a pioneer in this field. She spent many years identifying the magnitude of the problem in prisons, hospitals, factories, offices and schools. She also studied the relationship between pre-menstrual symptoms and crime, alcoholism and drug abuse. Quite a few of her studies are mentioned later on in the text, as they served as a starting point for our own research. Dr Dalton supports the theory that pre-menstrually low levels of the hormone progesterone are present. Her treatment consists largely of progesterone supplementation.

During the 1970s and 80s there were many attempts to identify a hormonal abnormality – a deficiency in women with PMS when compared with those who did not suffer. Many minor abnormalities, including elevated or decreased levels of progesterone, oestrogen and other hormones, were described in numerous small studies. However, no consistent pattern has emerged and the considered medical wisdom is that the vast majority of sufferers do not have a hormone excess or lack but are perhaps unduly sensitive to the normal swings in hormone levels that occur throughout the menstrual cycle. To support this new concept there is some very good evidence that the most powerful hormonal treatments are highly effective in controlling PMS. The reason for this is that if you can switch off the ovaries then you lose the normal rise and fall of hormone production, abolish the menstrual cycle, cease having periods and thus prevent PMS. No ovaries equals no PMS. Of course you then have a whole host of other problems as a result of this type of treatment.

Other workers have tried to link different patterns of pre-menstrual symptoms with changes either in hormones or in body chemistry. Dr Guy Abraham, a leading researcher from the United States, has over the last twenty years looked in detail at the relationship between nutritional factors, hormone function and PMS. Certain patterns can sometimes be discerned, thus allowing a more rational use of dietary treatments, and sometimes drug or hormonal treatments.

These are covered in some detail later on and we also show the benefits we have obtained using a nutritional approach. Many family doctors and experts now agree that tackling dietary and lifestyle factors is the best first-line approach to treating PMS.

As you have probably gathered, despite the fact that the Pre-Menstrual Syndrome has been approached from many angles, confusion still exists on the subject. There are those schools who believe the condition should be treated with hormones, whilst others believe it is a psychological condition which should be treated with tranquillizers and anti-depressants.

As a group we haven't set out to prove whether it is in fact a physical or mental condition. *We know it is a real condition.* Instead, we approach it from the viewpoint that certain symptoms exist which may be overcome by making dietary changes and adjustments in lifestyles where necessary. Between us we have many years of experience and have been able to help tens of thousands of women around the world to overcome their premenstrual problems.

I aim to give you a good understanding of what happens to your body during your monthly cycle. I will then help you to identify what the symptoms may be due to and then, of course, how you can go about getting them sorted out.

2

FUNCTIONING
NORMALLY

THE NORMAL MENSTRUAL CYCLE

In order to understand what is going wrong with your menstrual cycle, it is important to have a fairly good understanding of what the normal menstrual cycle is.

The age at the onset of periods has been decreasing at a rate of three years per century. Periods begin between the tenth and sixteenth year in 95 per cent of European girls, and between the tenth and fifteenth year in American girls. The age at the onset of the menopause, when periods cease, has been increasing at a rate of three years per century as well. Menopause occurs between the ages of 40 and 55.

The menstrual cycle is a fertility cycle, a fascinating process that enables a woman to conceive a child. This cycle is repeated each month, and if fertilization does not occur the cycle ends with a menstrual period – the shedding of the lining of the womb in preparation for the next cycle. The cycle can vary in length from approximately 22 days up to 34 days. Anything between these numbers would be considered normal. The first day of bleeding, the day the period arrives, is referred to as the first day of the cycle.

THE ORGANS INVOLVED

There are specific organs which each play an important role in the menstrual cycle. They are designed to work together so that a woman can become pregnant and nourish the growing child throughout the nine months of pregnancy.

The uterus or womb, as it is more commonly known, is a hollow, pear-shaped muscular organ which is about three inches (7.5 cm) long in a non-pregnant woman. There are many layers of specialized muscle here which, as if by magic, can expand so that the uterus becomes many times its usual size during pregnancy. The growing child lives in the uterus until it is ready to be born.

The innermost layer of the uterus is a membrane called the endometrium. During the cycle it becomes filled with the blood supply which would be needed to nourish a pregnancy. If conception has not occurred the endometrium breaks down, and together with the blood leaves the uterus through the neck of the uterus, which is known as the cervix.

The cervix or neck of the womb is like a little ball towards the back of the vagina. It has a small opening which remains closed for most of the time. A few days before the egg is released by the ovary, the cervix begins to open. By the time the egg has left the ovary, the opening would have become wide enough to let the sperm swim up through it, in order to gain access to the egg.

For a few days each cycle, at the time of ovulation, the specialized cells in the cervix produce fertile cervical mucus, which allows the sperm to live during their journey to the uterus. At other times during the menstrual cycle the cervix produces infertile cervical mucus which prevents the sperm from surviving.

Once the menstrual blood passes through the cervix it flows into the vaginal canal, a four- to six-inch (10–15 cm) muscular tube which has the ability to widen during sexual intercourse and during labour. During intercourse the lining of the vaginal canal becomes engorged with blood. A slippery liquid is produced which is designed to make the experience of sexual intercourse more comfortable.

The two almond-shaped organs on either side of the uterus are called the ovaries. They contain thousands of immature eggs which are present in a baby girl even before birth! From puberty, usually, one egg will leave one ovary during each menstrual cycle. I say usually, as there are occasions when more than one egg becomes fertilized simultaneously, and multiple births result.

OVULATION

The process of the egg leaving the ovary is called ovulation. At about 12 to 16 days before menstruation, the ovary will release an egg. The egg is then usually picked up by one of the Fallopian tubes, which is where the egg and the sperm would meet if conception were to take place. The Fallopian tubes are a pair of very thin tubes, about four inches (10 cm) long, which are connected to each side of the uterus. The egg waits for the sperm in the Fallopian tube for between 12 and 24 hours. If no sperm arrive, the egg is then absorbed by the body. If the egg and the sperm do meet and join up, fertilization takes place, and the fertilized egg will then move down, over the next few days, into the uterus, where it becomes embedded in the lining. This fertilized egg then grows into a baby.

WHAT CONTROLS THE CYCLE?

It is important to understand that although we have looked at the various organs at work for us during the menstrual cycle, it is actually the brain that controls the ovaries. In fact, a particular part of the brain called the pituitary gland sends instructions to the ovaries to make them function. The pituitary gland will tell the ovaries when to produce eggs and release them. It also stimulates production by the ovaries of oestrogen and progesterone, two very special sex hormones. If no fertilization occurs, the pituitary gland will send a new signal for the ovaries to begin producing eggs again.

WHAT ACTUALLY HAPPENS DURING THE CYCLE?

Either just prior to your period arriving, or during your period, several eggs will begin to grow in the ovary. Each egg is surrounded by a sac which is called a follicle. The egg and the follicle grow together. The follicle produces oestrogen which, as you can see from the chart overleaf, is at its highest during the latter part of the first half of the cycle. Oestrogen is responsible for the production of fertile cervical mucus, the opening of the cervix to allow the sperm in to meet the eggs, and the building up of blood in the lining of the uterus, preparing for a fertilized egg.

The cervical mucus is usually very fertile indeed: it is reckoned that sperm can survive for as long as five days in the fertile cervical mucus, waiting for an egg to fertilize. The egg is released from the ovary anything from eight to 14 days from the first day of your cycle – the day your period begins. Ovulation tends to vary from person to person. Some women are aware that they are ovulating as they experience some short-lived pain or stinging sensations in the area of the right or left ovary.

The cells or follicle that protected the egg before it was released remain

THE NORMAL MENSTRUAL CYCLE

1 ⎤
   ⎟   *Period begins – lining of uterus comes away. Very little progesterone.*
2 ⎦   *Very little oestrogen.*

3 ⎤
4 ⎟
5 ⎟   *Eggs growing and follicles beginning to produce oestrogen.*
6 ⎟
7 ⎦   *Oestrogen levels rising.*

8 ⎤
9 ⎟
10 ⎟
11 ⎟
12 ⎟   *Oestrogen levels high, stimulating the lining of the uterus to*
13 ⎦   *thicken.*

14 ——   *Ovulation occurs approximately at this time. Oestrogen levels are high. Once the egg has left, the follicle begins producing progesterone.*

15
16
17

18 ⎤
19 ⎟   *Oestrogen and progesterone levels high.*
20 ⎟
21 ⎟
22 ⎟
23 ⎟
24 ⎟
25 ⎦

26 ⎤   *Both progesterone and oestrogen levels falling now that conception*
27 ⎟   *has not occurred.*
28 ⎦

8

in the ovary after the egg has left. The follicle develops into a special gland known as the corpus luteum. Whereas the cells of the follicle were producing large amounts of oestrogen during the first half of the cycle, after ovulation they begin to produce the other important sex hormone, progesterone.

Progesterone is an important hormone at the beginning of pregnancy as it is responsible for producing infertile mucus, preventing sperm and other substances from harming a pregnancy. It is sometimes known as the pregnancy protecting hormone. It also closes the cervix and holds the lining of the uterus in place from ovulation until the next period begins, if fertilization has not taken place. Progesterone levels are sometimes low in women who suffer with PMS, and it has been demonstrated that balancing a woman's nutritional condition can raise the levels of progesterone again. This will be discussed later in the section on nutritional supplements on page 118.

After ovulation the body waits to see whether a pregnancy has occurred. Once it realizes that pregnancy has not occurred, the corpus luteum of the ovary stops working, and the levels of both oestrogen and progesterone fall. As progesterone has been holding the lining of the uterus in place, when this hormone level drops the lining of the uterus is then shed and a menstrual period occurs.

THE MAIN FACTS

Oestrogen controls the first half of the cycle until the egg leaves the ovary, and progesterone is in control of the cycle from the day the egg is released until the menstrual period begins.

The hormones produced by the ovaries have a profound effect on moods and behaviour – not surprising, since oestrogen is a stimulant of the nervous system. Low oestrogen levels cause depression, whereas high oestrogen levels can result in symptoms such as anxiety, irritability and nervous tension. The correct amount of oestrogen produces assertiveness, motivation and emotional stability. Progesterone, on the other hand, is a depressant, and has a calming effect. It is therefore obvious that for a woman to function normally throughout the menstrual cycle a proper balance of these hormones must be maintained.

I will be talking more about how the levels of oestrogen and progesterone are affected by a deficient nutritional state in Chapter 14 on vitamins and minerals, and our laboratory findings. Although it was previously thought that a woman had to take supplements of hormones in

HOW YOUR HORMONAL SYSTEM WORKS

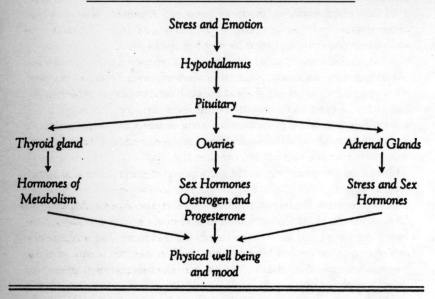

order to maintain her levels if she was deficient, it appears that this is not always so, as you will see.

EFFECTS OF NUTRITION
ON THE MENSTRUAL CYCLE

Nutrition affects the menstrual cycle in many ways. First, there are certain nutrients such as amino acids and vitamins that are necessary for the manufacture of brain hormones and the normal function of the pituitary gland, and which are also capable of influencing moods and behaviour.

Hormones are produced by the ovaries, adrenal glands and the thyroid gland. As already noted, the ovaries produce the sex hormones, oestrogen and progesterone. The adrenal glands produce both sex hormones and hormones related to stress. The thyroid gland produces its own hormones that control the body's rate of metabolism. These three glands – the ovaries, adrenals and thyroid – are all in turn controlled by a part of the brain, the pituitary which, if you like, is the conductor of the hormonal orchestra. It in turn is sensitive to a part of the brain called the hypothalamus which also influences appetite, temperature control and the 24-hour 'biological clock' that controls our eating and sleeping rhythms. It also contains another 'clock' that controls the 28-day menstrual cycle. Finally, it in turn is influenced by levels of stress and emotion. Thus it is that external stress and emotional factors can influence hormonal factors, and ultimately, one's physical sense of well-being and mood.

When an imbalanced diet exists or there are nutritional deficiencies the whole system may become disturbed or more sensitive. If there is a severe reduction in calorie (kj) intake and the body weight falls to an unhealthy level, the function of the pituitary gland will decrease and periods may cease altogether, or may continue but without ovulation. This is nature's way of protecting a woman from becoming pregnant when in an unhealthy state – a rather drastic form of contraception!

The hormones from the pituitary gland, thyroid gland, ovaries and adrenal gland all appear to be influenced slightly by the type of diet you eat, the balance of certain nutrients, exercise and stress. Vitamin B6, vitamin C, zinc, magnesium and other nutrients are subtly involved in the way in which the body responds to or processes the hormones that relate to the normal menstrual cycle. Making sure there is an adequate supply of these essential nutrients from the diet or from the use of supplements is one way to help combat PMS.

Finally, physical and emotional stress can have a powerful effect upon the menstrual cycle. For example, excessive or severe physical exercise, if continued on a regular basis, may cause the pituitary to 'switch off' the ovaries. Thus periods cease and the levels of the sex hormone oestrogen may fall. Such women put themselves at risk of fractures and thinning of the bones – osteoporosis. Emotional stress, such as the worry of becoming pregnant from having unprotected sexual intercourse, can itself lead to the delay or the missing of a period, which in turn causes increased worry and stress – not an uncommon experience at some time in one's life.

So a healthy diet and the avoidance of physical and mental stresses play an important part in health, and especially in the control of Pre-Menstrual Syndrome.

3

PMS DEFINED

PMS, or Pre-Menstrual Syndrome, is the term used to describe a collection of physical and mental symptoms that occur before a period starts and cease with or shortly after the arrival of a period.

WHEN DO SYMPTOMS BEGIN AND END?

- Most commonly symptoms begin from a week to a few days before menstruation begins, and then diminish as the period begins.

- Sometimes symptoms occur at the time of ovulation (mid cycle), then disappear until a few days pre-menstrually, when they recur until the onset of the period.

- Symptoms may begin at the time of ovulation, around the middle of the cycle, gradually increasing in severity until the period begins. It is not uncommon for symptoms to persist to the first day or two of the period.

WHAT IS THE DIFFERENCE BETWEEN PRE-MENSTRUAL SYNDROME AND PRE-MENSTRUAL TENSION?

- Pre-Menstrual Tension was the original name given to the collection of symptoms relating to tension and anxiety first reported by Dr Frank in the 1930s. Thus the condition became known as 'PMT'.

- Further research was done, particularly by Dr Dalton, who went on to discover further types of symptoms. She renamed the condition Pre-Menstrual Syndrome (PMS).

THE MOST COMMON PMS SYMPTOMS

Have a look at these symptoms. You might be surprised to realize that they are all associated with Pre-Menstrual Syndrome.

Nervous tension	Agoraphobia	Hayfever	Thoughts of
Mood swings	Bad breath	Fatigue	suicide
Irritability	Sensitivity to	Confusion	Sensitivity to
Anxiety	light	Forgetfulness	noise
Depression	Disorientation	Crying	Excessive thirst
Headache	Restlessness	Dizziness	Hostility
Migraine	Mouth ulcers	Tremors and	Sugar cravings
Insomnia	Acne	shakes	
Swollen breasts	Backache	Fainting	Weight gain
Tender/sore breasts	Heart poundings	Asthma	
Swollen abdomen	Cramp pains	Loss of interest	Diarrhoea
Bloated feelings	Wind	in sex	Cystitis
Craving for food	Generalized aches	Constipation	
Swelling of	Increased physical	Clumsiness	Boils
extremities	activity	Eczema	Hives
Heavy aching legs	Restless legs	Painful joints	Swollen ankles

JUST KNOWING THAT IT IS PMS

We are often told by patients that just knowing they have an identifiable, not to mention treatable, condition brings much relief in itself. It was a real surprise to me initially to discover women in all walks of life, with varying educational backgrounds, who were under the impression that their symptoms were in one of the following categories:

- All part of being a woman.
- Part of the ageing process.

- Early senile dementia.

- A psychological problem.

- A character fault.

- Schizophrenia.

The chances are that you may have been under an illusion that you fit in to one of these categories. I have lost count of the numbers of women who describe themselves as 'Jekyll and Hyde', i.e. two quite separate people during their menstrual cycle. They all seem to be acutely aware of the change as it occurs some time after ovulation. To a woman, they feel quite powerless to overcome the symptoms.

THE DIFFERENCE BETWEEN PMS AND PERIOD PAINS

Characteristic	PMS	Period pains
1. Time of onset	3–14 days before period	One day before and/or on first day or two of period
2. Improvement	Approximately the onset of the period	Some time during or at the end of the period
3. After childbirth	Symptoms worsen	Symptoms improve

4

THE MAKING OF PMS

There are a number of factors that may cause or contribute to PMS symptoms. It is very important to examine these thoroughly in order to get the situation into perspective.

GYNAECOLOGICAL OR HORMONAL PROBLEMS

If you have been experiencing problems for some time it is important to consult your doctor for a full check-up. Certainly if you have symptoms that are persistent all month through, there may be other complications present. Here is a small checklist for you to look at to see whether there need be cause for any concern:

- Heavy or irregular periods.
- Abdominal pain.
- Excessive weight gain or weight loss.
- Facial hair growth.
- Persistent severe headaches.
- Current vaginal discharge, soreness or irritation.
- Breast lumps or tenderness throughout the menstrual cycle.
- Milky discharge from the nipples.

If any of these are a current problem it would be advisable to get them checked out, for peace of mind if nothing else. You will then establish whether you have other medical problems as well as PMS, or pure PMS.

FACTORS IN THE CAUSATION OF PMS

1. Difficulty with relationships.

2. Problems with work.

3. Problem children to cope with.

4. Disturbed night's sleep.

5. Financial difficulties causing friction and worries.

6. Strained relations with husband or partner.

7. Inadequate or incorrect diet.

8. Environmental pollutants.

9. Social poisons.

10. Oral contraceptive pill.

11. Increasing age, especially age 30–40.

12. After childbirth.

13. Lack of exercise.

14. Operations and physical illnesses.

EXAMINING PMS SYMPTOMS

WHAT ACTUALLY CAUSES PMS

In Chapter 2, 'Functioning Normally', hormonal changes throughout the menstrual cycle were described. Whilst major disturbance of hormone levels is not the sole explanation for PMS, certain variations in hormone levels or sensitivity to hormones may well be part of the cause. This in turn can be influenced by stress, dietary factors and nutritional state.

If you are confused about the cause of PMS, don't worry, as most medical scientists and researchers are just as perplexed. Dr Guy Abraham, former Professor of Obstetrics and Gynaecology at the University of California in Los Angeles, has attempted to unravel the causation of PMS by dividing the symptoms into four groups, as detailed below. This somewhat artificial classification does help us to develop possible explanations as to the cause of different aspects of PMS symptoms. Disturbances in the levels of oestrogen and progesterone have been described in some sufferers with different types of PMS, but these are not universal changes. Furthermore, many women will experience symptoms from more than one sub-group.

PMS A (ANXIETY)

This is the most common sub-group. Symptoms are recorded in about 80 per cent of sufferers. The symptoms in this group are:

Nervous tension.
Mood swings.
Irritability.
Anxiety.

PMS H (HYDRATION)

This is the second sub-group. It is estimated that symptoms occur in 60 per cent of sufferers. The symptoms in the sub-group are as follows:

Weight gain.
Swelling of extremities.
Breast tenderness.
Abdominal bloating.

PMS C (CRAVING)

This is the third sub-group. Symptoms probably occur in 40 per cent of sufferers. There are six symptoms in this sub-group:

Headache.
Craving for sweets.
Increased appetite.
Heart pounding.
Fatigue.
Dizziness or fainting.

PMS D (DEPRESSION)

Of all four sub-groups, this is the one least commonly found on its own. Perhaps 20 per cent of sufferers have PMS D. There are five symptoms in this category:

Depression.
Forgetfulness.
Crying.
Confusion.
Insomnia.

Each group seems to have different factors involved, except that inadequate diet and stress can be common to all of them. Although some women only suffer with one sub-group of symptoms, it is just as common to be suffering from any combination of sub-groups at the same time. Many severe sufferers seem to have symptoms in all four sub-groups initially.

In the next four chapters I will examine in greater detail each one of these sub-groups of symptoms and look at how the symptoms affected the lives of some of the women who contacted the Women's Nutritional Advisory Service. Rather than describing how PMS might affect various aspects of your life, I decided that the subject might become more alive if it was talked about by sufferers themselves. I have selected patients whose symptoms span a broad spectrum of the Pre-Menstrual Syndrome. By looking into their lives you may well recognize familiar situations.

5

ANXIOUS, IRRITABLE AND UPTIGHT

PMS A (ANXIETY)

The main symptoms of PMS A are nervous tension, anxiety, irritability and mood swings, beginning as early as two weeks before the period and becoming progressively worse as the period approaches.

There are several possible factors, both hormonal and dietary, that might cause pre-menstrual anxiety. Some doctors think that an excess of the hormone oestrogen or an increased sensitivity to it may trigger changes in brain chemistry, resulting in anxiety. The average diet, high in fat and relatively low in fibre, can increase the levels of this hormone. Also, high levels of oestrogen slow down the rate at which the stimulant caffeine is broken down by the liver. This is why some women become more sensitive to tea and coffee when they are pregnant or when taking the oral contraceptive pill.

A lack of vitamin B and possibly the mineral magnesium can also cause changes in the chemistry of the nervous system that can aggravate feelings of anxiety and irritability. Interestingly it seems that some women (and men) who are prone to anxiety and panic attacks are more sensitive to caffeine and genuinely have a more sensitive body metabolism which makes them very susceptible to the effects of a lack of vitamin B or magnesium.

A comparison of caffeine consumption in Chinese nurses and workers in a tea factory revealed a strong association between increased caffeine consumption and the severity of pre-menstrual symptoms. We conducted our own survey in the United Kingdom with *Fitness* magazine which was published in 1992. 377 women took part. Caffeine consumption was

19

nearly two and a half times higher in PMS sufferers compared with non-sufferers.

On average a mug of tea contains 100 to 130 mg and a mug of coffee between 150 and 250 mg of caffeine. In excess of 250 mg of caffeine can produce symptoms of anxiety, irritability, headache, increased passage of urine and a shaking feeling. Insomnia and palpitations can also occur. It is therefore advisable that these ever popular beverages are limited to just one or two cups or mugs per day and that caffeine-free alternatives are used. More details about these can be found on pages 107-108.

A final and important factor is hyperventilation. This mouthful simply means over breathing. Often when one becomes anxious it is natural to increase the rate and depth of respiration. This provides more oxygen to the bloodstream but also removes more of the waste gas carbon dioxide. This lack of carbon dioxide causes a change in body chemistry which can actually aggravate or cause a variety of symptoms, including numbness and tingling of the fingers, hands and around the mouth, muscle cramps, headaches, light-headedness, increased anxiety, physical and mental fatigue and confusion. The solution is to relax, reduce the rate and depth of breathing and if symptoms are severe to breathe in and out of a paper bag for several minutes. Where these symptoms chronically occur, formal advice and breathing exercises may need to be given by a physiotherapist or psychologist.

ABOUT THE SYMPTOMS

The symptoms in PMS A can at least be disturbing, and at worst feel like a tidal wave of personality change. They are amongst the most common symptoms in PMS.

A staggering 97 per cent of women in our survey of 1000 PMS patients, who were suffering moderately to severely, complained that they suffered to some degree with irritability pre-menstrually, 73 per cent of them with severe irritability, 96 per cent reported mood swings, 62 per cent severe, while 95 per cent reported nervous tension, 60 per cent severe, and 91 per cent reported anxiety, 54 per cent severe.

Degree of irritability suffered out of a sample of 1000 women				
Not Affected	Mild	Moderate	Severe	Total Affected
2.5%	3.2%	20.8%	73.5% -	97.5%

As you can imagine, the implications of these figures are fairly devastating. No wonder so many women report Jekyll and Hyde syndrome! Let us look more closely at how PMS A affected the lives of some of our patients.

PMS HITS HOME!

Many women were also reporting wild feelings of violence and aggression pre-menstrually. Their nervous tension seemed to reach uncontrollable peaks, at which time they would lash out at children and husbands or boyfriends. To a woman, they reported that this behaviour was uncharacteristic of them, and that it was having disastrous effects on their families.

The chart below shows to what degree violent and aggressive feelings were a problem. We were very concerned indeed by the result of our research.

Just under 80 per cent of the women studied felt violent or aggressive pre-menstrually. This obviously had serious repercussions on their partners, and on their children in particular.

Sample of 1000 women who admitted being violent/aggressive whilst suffering from PMS				
Not Affected	Once	More Than Once	More Than Six Times	Total Affected
20.6%	4.7%	27.7%	47.0% -	79.4%

" Pauline's Story "

Pauline experienced extreme violent and aggressive feelings pre-menstrually. She actually used to strike her husband and her daughter. She relates her experiences here very frankly.

Pauline is a 35-year-old mother and housewife who has had PMS since she was 13 years old.

'I used to be able to cope when I was in my teens but as I became older, my symptoms became really dreadful. I used to feel groggy for the whole week before my period. I had terrible migraine headaches and my head felt like it was full of cotton wool. Towards the end I'd have to spend the last few days in bed as I had no energy. I also had severe insomnia, dizziness and forgetfulness.

Eventually I started hitting my one-year-old daughter. I knew it was wrong but I couldn't control myself. I even hit my husband. I tried to carry on with life pre-menstrually but the very thought of going out of the house sent me into fits of the shakes. I was very frightened of meeting people. In fact, I was terrified!

I was given so many treatments for PMS. First my doctor prescribed different types of pill. Then I had Valium and I wasn't sleeping. That's when the depression started. Then I had anti-depressants. I felt like a junkie with my "uppers and downers".

Hormone treatment made me feel worse, and so finally I was referred to a psychologist who prescribed narcosis (i.e. being sedated and put to sleep) which lasted three days. This failed to help, and so the psychologist suggested giving me a course of ECT. I was very frightened, really desperate, I felt as though I was cracking up. It wasn't any wonder that my marriage split up. I even attempted suicide.

I just felt like I wanted to shut the door and be on my own, and yet I didn't want to be on my own, it was most peculiar.

I disliked myself

I just felt a mess pre-menstrually. An absolute mess. I really didn't like myself at all. The thing was that in my teens I could cope with it, because it was every few months and only for a day or two before my period. I was slimmer then and I had long blonde hair. As I got older and had Emma I just felt like a slob because everything had gone, everything had dropped, my skin was really terrible and itchy and my hair was greasy.

Relationships

Steve and I had been married for ten years before he started retaliating. So he'd put up with me for a long time. He'd put up with a lot. I've thrown things down the stairs at him and even hit him right across the face in front of our daughter. He's 5 ft 10 ins (1 m 75 cm) and quite reserved and easy-going usually.

I can remember a day when he happened to mention the curtains I'd just hand-sewn were not wide enough. I flew into a rage and kicked him, then flew upstairs and cried. When I came down we started arguing and fighting over something else. That's when he started hitting back.

My terrified little daughter

Emma was a wonderful, active child and began talking by eight months. By twelve months she would answer back and be deliberately defiant. I could only put up with her for so long pre-menstrually and then I'd hit her. I knew I shouldn't have done that. I realize it now because she was only twelve months old. She's been smacked much more than she should have been.

She was growing up to be a frightened little girl. She just didn't know which way her mummy was going to be. She was very frightened of me, so much so, she didn't want to be left alone in the house with me, especially when I was pre-menstrual. That is a dreadful way for a child to be.

23

PRE-MENSTRUAL SYNDROME QUESTIONNAIRE

Name: _Pauline Solent_   Age: _35_   Height: _5' 5"_   Weight: _9st 10lb_

MARITAL STATUS: Single ____   Married _✓_   Divorced ____   Widowed ____
(Please tick where applicable)

PRESENT CONTRACEPTION: None _✓_   Pill ____   I.U.D. ____   Other ____

  Your periods come every _31–33_ days   Your periods last _7_ days

  Your periods are: Light ____   Moderate ____   Heavy _✓_

  Number of Pregnancies: _1_   Number of Miscarriages: ____

Birth weight of children:
  1st child _6lb 4oz_   2nd child ____   3rd child ____   4th child ____

SYMPTOMS	WEEK AFTER PERIOD (Fill in 3 days after period)				WEEK BEFORE PERIOD (Fill in 2-3 days before period)			
	None	Mild	Moderate	Severe	None	Mild	Moderate	Severe
PMS - A								
Nervous Tension				✓				✓
Mood Swings	✓							✓
Irritability			✓					✓
Anxiety			✓					✓
PMS - H								
Weight Gain	✓				✓			
Swelling of Extremities	✓				✓			
Breast Tenderness	✓							✓
Abdominal Bloating	✓							✓
PMS - C								
Headache				✓				✓
Craving for Sweets	✓							✓
Increased Appetite	✓				✓			
Heart Pounding	✓							✓
Fatigue			✓					✓
Dizziness or Fainting			✓					✓
PMS - D								
Depression				✓				✓
Forgetfulness	✓							✓
Crying			✓					✓
Confusion	✓							✓
Insomnia				✓				✓
OTHER SYMPTOMS								
Loss of Sexual Interest				✓				✓
Disorientation	✓				✓			
Clumsiness	✓							✓
Tremors/Shakes	✓							✓
Thoughts of Suicide		✓						✓
Agoraphobia			✓					✓
Increased Physical Activity	✓				✓			
Heavy/Aching Legs	✓				✓			
Generalized Aches	✓							✓
Bad Breath	✓				✓			
Sensitivity to Music/Light	✓							✓
Excessive Thirst	✓							✓

FOLLOW UP
PRE-MENSTRUAL SYNDROME QUESTIONNAIRE

Name: Pauline Solent   Age: 35   Height: 5' 5"   Weight: 9st 2lb

MARITAL STATUS: Single ____ Married _√_ Divorced ____ Widowed ____
(Please tick where applicable)

PRESENT CONTRACEPTION: None _√_ Pill ____ I.U.D. ____ Other ____

   Your periods come every 31–33 days   Your periods last 5–7 days

   Your periods are: Light ____ Moderate _√_ Heavy ____

SYMPTOMS

	WEEK AFTER PERIOD (Fill in 3 days after period)				WEEK BEFORE PERIOD (Fill in 2-3 days before period)			
	None	Mild	Moderate	Severe	None	Mild	Moderate	Severe
PMS - A								
Nervous Tension	√				√			
Mood Swings	√				√			
Irritability	√				√			
Anxiety	√				√			
PMS - H								
Weight Gain	√				√			
Swelling of Extremities	√				√			
Breast Tenderness	√				√			
Abdominal Bloating	√				√			
PMS - C								
Headache	√				√			
Craving for Sweets	√				√			
Increased Appetite	√				√			
Heart Pounding	√				√			
Fatigue	√				√			
Dizziness or Fainting	√				√			
PMS - D								
Depression	√				√			
Forgetfulness	√				√			
Crying	√				√			
Confusion	√				√			
Insomnia	√				√			
OTHER SYMPTOMS								
Loss of Sexual Interest	√				√			
Disorientation	√				√			
Clumsiness	√				√			
Tremors/Shakes	√				√			
Thoughts of Suicide	√				√			
Agoraphobia	√				√			
Increased Physical Activity	√				√			
Heavy/Aching Legs	√				√			
Generalized Aches	√				√			
Bad Breath	√				√			
Sensitivity to Music/Light	√				√			
Excessive Thirst	√				√			

Hormone treatment

After my overdose my doctor decided to try me on a hormone treatment. Shortly after I started on hormones I developed very severe breast tenderness. My breasts literally stood out and they were so sore and uncomfortable. I kept taking them for two months but the problem just intensified. I ended up taking pain killers every day to try to ease the pain.

I decided to stop taking the hormone treatment but that was easier said than done. I had awful withdrawal symptoms even though I came off them gradually. First I took two per day, then one, then every other day. The symptoms were so awful and, Oh my head! I've never known anything like it. I couldn't bear to put a foot down in front of me. The food cravings I had were unbelievable. I vowed I would never take another tablet for the rest of my life.

Relief at last

I read about the Women's Nutritional Advisory Service in the local newspaper. I was at my wits' end at the time at the thought of spending another weekend in bed with terrible sweats and shakes. I felt like it was the last resort before I accepted the ECT. Fortunately, they managed to sort me out in the first five days, it was unbelievable!'

Pauline suffered very severely with PMS, to the point where she was at times a danger to herself and certainly a liability to her family. Her whole life revolved around her pre-menstrual symptoms. She was, sadly, unable to lead a normal life and on the point of having psychiatric treatment, ECT, when she contacted us. (ECT, electroconvulsive therapy, electric shock treatment, kills brain cells and these do not regenerate.)

The chart from her first questionnaire has been copied on page 24. This she completed when she first contacted us. You will notice that quite a few symptoms in each category were severe pre-menstrually. She was, in fact, suffering with all four categories of PMS listed. However, most of the symptoms in PMS A, the first category, were so severe that they were still present the week after her period. We soon discovered that this was largely due to her nutritional state and her diet. I will explain this more fully in the Diet section on page 142. She admits herself that she responded exceedingly quickly to a change in diet and nutritional supplements of vitamins and minerals.

Previous diet

'I *used to drink nine or 10 cups of tea per day and I used a lot of salt* both in my cooking and at the table. I ate lots of convenience foods like pre-packed pies and tinned foods and I ate a fair amount of cheese, milk and wholemeal (wholewheat) bread. Also, I could easily eat four or five biscuits a day.

New diet

I think the diet suggested by the Women's Nutritional Advisory Service is wonderful. I found it a little difficult at first but I think that's because my head was so peculiar pre-menstrually that I couldn't take it all in.

When the programme arrived I drove to my mum's and we sat down together and read through it so that we understood it fully. She then came with me to the supermarket and I bought lots of leeks, fresh vegetables and fruit, salad and fish. I had to cut out wholewheat and all foods containing yeast. I was given lists of foods to avoid and lists of food to concentrate on. I eat loads of fresh food now and feel wonderful. My friends all know I'm on a special diet. It's become a way of life.'

Pauline's follow-up questionnaire after six months on page 25 looks dramatically different. All her pre-menstrual symptoms are gone completely.

End result

'I don't have any symptoms any more. My life has changed dramatically. I feel much more at ease and I never shout, unless I am very angry.

My agoraphobia has gone completely. I can go out with confidence and I feel great in myself. I can do all the things I couldn't do before. I can go anywhere.

Steve and I get on really well now, so much so we are even planning to have another baby, which I could never have coped with before. I had no intention of having any more children, in fact I'd given away all the baby equipment. I am truly delighted with the results of my programme. My husband thinks it's wonderful too.'

From a letter Pauline sent at the end of her programme you can tell she is now coping with life and feels normal again.

Dear Maryon,

I am very fit now and I have just spent a hectic week in London with my six-year-old daughter – who is a handful. I feel marvellous. She's been better as I have practically put her on my diet (except she does have some sweets), and she watches my diet.

Thanks again for giving me my life back after 20 years.

Yours ever so grateful
Pauline Solent

" Ruth's Story "

Ruth was another victim of violent and aggressive feelings which she acted on pre-menstrually. Classically, she didn't experience any of these feelings once her period arrived.

Ruth is a 39-year-old who is a housewife and a mother of two children. Her PMS began after the birth of her first baby, although she feels it may have been simmering beforehand.

'PMS totally changed my character when I had it, and I had it for half my life. It began two weeks before my period, sometimes more. It would disappear on the first day of my period and I immediately felt a sense of relief. Then a week after my period it began to build up again.

I became very irritable, very tired, snappy and aggressive, which is not a bit what I'm like normally. I would shout at my husband, literally scream at him. I think I still have sore throats as a result. I used to go to my room and have a screaming fit to keep it to myself. But people would aggravate me easily. Obviously when you have small children they tend to get on your nerves when you are tired. I felt like a lump of lead at the time and I know I had very little patience with my older daughter who was my only child when it was at its worst. She suffered, I'm sure. I would scream at her and hit her at times which was very upsetting for me afterwards because I know a child of seven couldn't possibly understand.

I vowed it wouldn't happen next month

Although my husband was understanding and sympathetic, it's very difficult to have a normal relationship with someone when they are aggressive and not well. There is no doubt about the fact that the presence of PMS symptoms placed a strain on our marriage.

I suppose everybody has irritating habits and normally I would just take them in my stride. But at PMS times my husband would aggravate me to

28

the point where I'd scream at him. Unfortunately it was over stupid, insignificant things.

Very often I'd take it out on the children instead of my husband. This was because I knew he had such high standards of self-discipline and I think he felt that I ought to have been able to do something about my own behaviour. I always vowed that next month I was jolly well going to, it was mind over matter etc., but it never seemed to work.

I hated myself

When pre-menstrual I felt I was awful, I really hated myself. When I started hitting my daughter, I felt like I had really failed myself. I felt like a worm. Really dreadful. I cannot explain how I felt. My usual philosophy is that if children are treated right they respond and they are not naughty. I tried to explain to my doctor but he didn't understand. I remember shouting at him "you don't understand" but he just threw his hands up in horror and walked out of the surgery.

My daughter locked herself away from me

I think my daughter was quite frightened of me actually. I am normally placid but of course I wasn't, as my symptoms were occurring more often than not when I was at my worst.

The problem would usually begin over a trivial matter which now I would brush aside or cope with calmly. Then I would just feel so tight inside and, of course, it would then become a big thing. Of course with children if you build it up they build it up also, and it all gets out of hand. I would sometimes grip her and shake her, poor girl. It was a dreadful way to treat a child. She would often go off and lock herself in her bedroom because she was afraid of me.

I never did her any bad damage, but it was awful to me as I would never normally strike a child. I don't agree with bashing children when they are naughty, particularly as she probably wasn't even that naughty. It just got out of hand.

Previous treatments

The first time I went to the doctor about my PMS, and I have been to several doctors about it over the years, it was thought a good idea for me to take the Pill to remove the "tension" beforehand. This was after the birth of my first child, about 14 years ago. The Pill caused me awful headaches and I had to come off it.

PRE-MENSTRUAL SYNDROME QUESTIONNAIRE

Name: Ruth Sears   Age: 39   Height: 5' 11"   Weight: 12st

MARITAL STATUS: Single _____   Married _✓_   Divorced _____   Widowed _____
(Please tick where applicable)

PRESENT CONTRACEPTION: None_____   Pill_____   I.U.D. _✓_   Other_____

   Your periods come every ___28___ days   Your periods last ___5___ days

   Your periods are: Light_____   Moderate _✓_   Heavy_____

   Number of Pregnancies: ___3___   Number of Miscarriages: ___1___

Birth weight of children:
1st child _7lb 15oz_ 2nd child _8lb 10oz_ 3rd child_____ 4th child_____

SYMPTOMS	WEEK AFTER PERIOD (Fill in 3 days after period)				WEEK BEFORE PERIOD (Fill in 2-3 days before period)			
	None	Mild	Moderate	Severe	None	Mild	Moderate	Severe
PMS - A								
Nervous Tension	✓							✓
Mood Swings	✓							✓
Irritability	✓							✓
Anxiety	✓						✓	
PMS - H								
Weight Gain	✓						✓	
Swelling of Extremities	✓				✓			
Breast Tenderness	✓				✓			
Abdominal Bloating	✓						✓	
PMS - C								
Headache	✓				✓			
Craving for Sweets	✓							✓
Increased Appetite	✓							✓
Heart Pounding	✓				✓			
Fatigue	✓							✓
Dizziness or Fainting	✓				✓			
PMS - D								
Depression	✓							✓
Forgetfulness	✓							✓
Crying	✓				✓			
Confusion	✓							✓
Insomnia	✓				✓			
OTHER SYMPTOMS								
Loss of Sexual Interest	✓							✓
Disorientation	✓						✓	
Clumsiness	✓						✓	
Tremors/Shakes	✓				✓			
Thoughts of Suicide	✓				✓			
Agoraphobia	✓				✓			
Increased Physical Activity	✓				✓			
Heavy/Aching Legs	✓				✓			
Generalized Aches	✓				✓			
Bad Breath	✓				✓			
Sensitivity to Music/Light	✓				✓			
Excessive Thirst	✓				✓			

I realized I couldn't continue to suffer, by which time my original doctor had left the practice. The new doctor prescribed vitamin B6. He wanted to try the natural approach first before prescribing progesterone. Although I thought that the vitamin B6 was helping at first, it didn't make the slightest difference to my symptoms.

I saw a specialist who examined me thoroughly and could find nothing physically wrong. He said it was a hormonal imbalance and prescribed hormone treatment. I was never very happy about taking hormones, I would rather have taken more natural things. They did help my symptoms though, to the point where I could function to some degree. But PMS reared its ugly head again. It would pop up now and then. It was not fully quashed. Life wasn't what I would describe as being bearable, but it was more under control than before.

My husband then read an article in the newspaper about the nutritional programme for PMS being so successful and suggested I follow that up.'

Ruth struggled for 14 years with her symptoms. Again, it affected a large portion of her life. She admits her family suffered a great deal because of her behaviour pre-menstrually. And in common with all the other sufferers mentioned, she was unable to control herself. When her period began all her symptoms went.

She suffered severely with three categories of PMS: PMS A, the nervous and uptight symptoms, PMS C, craving for sweet foods etc., and PMS D, particularly depression, confusion and forgetfulness. She had tried many treatments before to help ease her symptoms, but she was unable to control the situation. Long-term hormone treatment did help to ease things a bit, but she was unhappy taking them.

Her first chart is opposite.

Diet helped

'I really had no idea that diet was an important factor in controlling PMS. I thought it was a question of hormone balance being wrong. And the only way to put it right was to put in more hormones, the right kind of hormones, rather than eat different things.

I used to drink quite a bit of coffee, add lots of salt to my food, and I had a lot of sugary foods. I used to try to eat a high fibre and low fat diet because I was always trying to get my weight down. I did have a weakness for chocolates and biscuits, in fact I used to crave them especially pre-menstrually.

31

FOLLOW UP
PRE-MENSTRUAL SYNDROME QUESTIONNAIRE

Name: Ruth Sears   Age: 39   Height: 5' 11"   Weight: 12st

MARITAL STATUS: Single _____   Married _√_   Divorced _____   Widowed _____
(Please tick where applicable)

PRESENT CONTRACEPTION: None_____   Pill_____   I.U.D. _√_   Other_____

Your periods come every __28__ days   Your periods last __5__ days

Your periods are: Light_____   Moderate __√__   Heavy_____

SYMPTOMS	WEEK AFTER PERIOD (Fill in 3 days after period)				WEEK BEFORE PERIOD (Fill in 2-3 days before period)			
	None	Mild	Moderate	Severe	None	Mild	Moderate	Severe
PMS - A								
Nervous Tension	√				√			
Mood Swings	√				√			
Irritability	√				√			
Anxiety	√				√			
PMS - H								
Weight Gain	√				√			
Swelling of Extremities	√				√			
Breast Tenderness	√						√	
Abdominal Bloating	√	√			√			
PMS - C								
Headache	√				√			
Craving for Sweets	√				√			
Increased Appetite	√				√			
Heart Pounding	√				√			
Fatigue	√	√			√			
Dizziness or Fainting	√				√			
PMS - D								
Depression	√				√			
Forgetfulness	√				√			
Crying	√				√			
Confusion	√				√			
Insomnia	√				√			
OTHER SYMPTOMS								
Loss of Sexual Interest	√				√			
Disorientation	√				√			
Clumsiness	√				√			
Tremors/Shakes	√				√			
Thoughts of Suicide	√				√			
Agoraphobia	√				√			
Increased Physical Activity	√				√			
Heavy/Aching Legs	√				√			
Generalized Aches	√				√			
Bad Breath	√				√			
Sensitivity to Music/Light	√				√			
Excessive Thirst	√				√			

I read an article in the newspaper about the Women's Nutritional Advisory Service dietary recommendations, so I was semi-prepared when I received my programme. Being asked to cut out grains shocked me a bit. It was the most complicated part of the diet, I found, as so many things contain wheat.

I did stick to the diet to the letter for the first three months. I even had a special meal prepared when we attended a formal dinner. No one asked why, and I didn't want to mention the reason. They were all very discreet about it. It didn't cause a problem.

My symptoms completely vanished on the programme. It was absolute magic. Even my long-standing problem of thrush cleared up when I was avoiding wheat and foods containing yeast.

I am back on all the usual foods now. I no longer have the intense sweet cravings and I feel I know where to draw the line. I still take Optivite, a vitamin supplement which I think is marvellous, and my symptoms haven't returned.

I'm delighted to say that my life has been transformed since starting on the programme. I followed the suggested diet very closely for six months and took the recommended vitamin and mineral supplements. In fact, I still take the supplements but have been able to moderate my diet. It seems amazing to me that such strong, violent symptoms could be controlled by changing my diet and taking some vitamin pills.'

Her follow-up questionnaire (opposite) reflects her progress. Most symptoms are completely under control. Just a bit of mild breast tenderness pre-menstrually remains.

End result

'Since undertaking the nutritional programme to overcome my PMS, I can honestly say my symptoms have disappeared. I think they have really vanished, like absolute magic. I am overwhelmed by it. My life is now back to normal. There is no comparison in me now. I am a completely different woman. Back to what I was before.'

Ruth's letter to me at the end of her programme was interesting as she points out that it is sometimes genuinely difficult to come off treatment – even it it isn't really working. Trying a new approach does often involve courage, especially when so many other treatments have failed previously.

Dear Maryon,

I am enclosing my follow-up questionnaire and must take the opportunity to tell you how absolutely the course has changed my life. I couldn't have believed that just vitamins, minerals and a change of diet could have such a dramatic impact.

Having had quite severe symptoms it was an act of courage and determination to break off the progesterone treatment and step into the blue on your programme. I'm glad I did.

Ruth Sears

Here is another example of how PMS A symptoms affected the life of a young single woman, who was also diagnosed as having irritable bowel syndrome.

Nadine is a 25-year-old single woman who works as an advertising executive. She has been suffering with PMS since she was 15 years of age and feels that her life has been pretty disrupted as a result.

" Nadine's Story "

'I felt trapped like a victim, trapped in the philosophy of being a woman and stuck with it. I was very fed up with the suffering every month, it was like being in a biological prison. I was very frightened.

PMS just meant misery to me, it made my life difficult and extremely unpleasant. That's the best way I can explain it. The fact that I had no idea what it was, made matters worse. From the age of 15 I was extremely unpleasant pre-menstrually, to my mother in particular. I would start shouting at her. I was very aggressive and argumentative before my period. Unfortunately, I wasn't aware of the pattern at the time.

My social life was affected by my symptoms and at work I just got a reputation for being an extremely rude person. In fact, previously at college I had been nicknamed "The Misery".

I used to take my frustrations out on my boyfriend. I'd lash out at him with my fists, then I would throw things around the room. That was the worst thing, feeling so aggressive and throwing things around. He would try to calm me down by cuddling me. He knew if he rode the storm that I would calm down eventually when my period came.

My tummy problems were so severe I was diagnosed by my doctor as having irritable bowel syndrome, caused by stress. I felt that that was a

34

very convenient diagnosis to make when he didn't really know what the problem was and he wanted to get rid of me. "Tell them it's stress and they'll go away."

I felt pretty awful. I tried to help myself by taking some vitamin B6, then I tried evening primrose oil and zinc, and finally my doctor prescribed progesterone suppositories. None of the treatments were successful, though.

It wasn't until I read articles in magazines about the work that the Women's Nutritional Advisory Service was doing that I came to realize that I was suffering from PMS. Up until then I was just aware that my symptoms were getting worse and worse and I didn't know what to do about them.'

Nadine is a young, single woman who has not had any children. Nevertheless, at the time she came to us she had been suffering with PMS symptoms for some 10 years. Her main problem areas were the tension and anxiety symptoms, and the swelling and bloating symptoms, as you can see from her chart overleaf.

Understandably, she was frightened about the effect that her ever-recurring symptoms had on her body and on her life. All areas of her life were disrupted because of her symptoms, and despite trying a series of treatments, both independently, and through her doctor, her symptoms showed no sign of easing off. The thought of going through her whole life suffering in this manner had been pretty uncomfortable to Nadine.

Diet

'My previous diet obviously wasn't right, in retrospect. I had a very bad stomach problem, in fact I was diagnosed as having irritable bowel disease. I had loads of unpleasant tests and was told that the condition was due to stress.

I used to get terrible diarrhoea and pain cramps in my tummy. The doctors told me to eat more bran, which I have since found out aggravates the condition.

I didn't know that diet could play such an important role. I did wonder sometimes though. I did a degree in Food Science and there was a small amount of information on the effects that diet could have on the body. Although I had my suspicions, I didn't know how to go about finding out more. I did try looking for papers but I didn't really find many and I didn't find anything to connect diet to PMS or my irritable bowel problem.

I used to eat up to four slices of wholemeal (wholewheat) bread per day

PRE-MENSTRUAL SYNDROME QUESTIONNAIRE

Name: Nadine Morris   Age: 25   Height: 5' 2"   Weight: 10st 4lb

MARITAL STATUS: Single __✓__ Married _____ Divorced _____ Widowed _____
(Please tick where applicable)

PRESENT CONTRACEPTION: None_____ Pill_____ I.U.D._____ Other __✓__

Your periods come every __27–35__ days   Your periods last __4–5__ days

   Your periods are: Light_____ Moderate __✓__ Heavy_____

   Number of Pregnancies: __1__   Number of Miscarriages: __1__

Birth weight of children:
1st child_____ 2nd child_____ 3rd child_____ 4th child_____

SYMPTOMS	WEEK AFTER PERIOD (Fill in 3 days after period)				WEEK BEFORE PERIOD (Fill in 2-3 days before period)			
	None	Mild	Moderate	Severe	None	Mild	Moderate	Severe
PMS - A								
Nervous Tension	✓							✓
Mood Swings	✓							✓
Irritability	✓							✓
Anxiety		✓						✓
PMS - H								
Weight Gain	✓						✓	
Swelling of Extremities	✓				✓			
Breast Tenderness	✓						✓	
Abdominal Bloating		✓						✓
PMS - C								
Headache	✓				✓			
Craving for Sweets	✓					✓		
Increased Appetite	✓					✓		
Heart Pounding	✓				✓			
Fatigue	✓				✓			
Dizziness or Fainting	✓				✓			
PMS - D								
Depression	✓				✓			
Forgetfulness	✓				✓			
Crying	✓					✓		
Confusion	✓				✓			
Insomnia	✓				✓			
OTHER SYMPTOMS								
Loss of Sexual Interest	✓				✓			
Disorientation	✓				✓			
Clumsiness		✓						✓
Tremors/Shakes	✓				✓			
Thoughts of Suicide	✓				✓			
Agoraphobia								
Increased Physical Activity		✓			✓			
Heavy/Aching Legs	✓				✓			
Generalized Aches	✓				✓			
Bad Breath	✓				✓			
Sensitivity to Music/Light	✓				✓			
Excessive Thirst	✓							✓

FOLLOW UP
PRE-MENSTRUAL SYNDROME QUESTIONNAIRE

Name: Nadine Morris   Age: 25   Height: 5' 2"   Weight: 9st 9lb

MARITAL STATUS: Single √   Married____   Divorced____   Widowed____
(Please tick where applicable)

PRESENT CONTRACEPTION: None____   Pill____   I.U.D.____   Other √

Your periods come every 28–35 days   Your periods last   4–5   days

Your periods are: Light_____   Moderate____ √   Heavy_____

SYMPTOMS	WEEK AFTER PERIOD (Fill in 3 days after period)				WEEK BEFORE PERIOD (Fill in 2-3 days before period)			
	None	Mild	Moderate	Severe	None	Mild	Moderate	Severe
PMS - A								
Nervous Tension	√				√			
Mood Swings	√				√			
Irritability	√				√			
Anxiety	√				√			
PMS - H								
Weight Gain	√				√			
Swelling of Extremities	√				√			
Breast Tenderness	√				√			
Abdominal Bloating	√				√			
PMS - C								
Headache	√				√			
Craving for Sweets	√				√			
Increased Appetite	√				√			
Heart Pounding	√				√			
Fatigue	√				√			
Dizziness or Fainting	√				√			
PMS - D								
Depression	√				√			
Forgetfulness	√				√			
Crying	√				√			
Confusion	√				√			
Insomnia	√				√			
OTHER SYMPTOMS								
Loss of Sexual Interest	√				√			
Disorientation	√				√			
Clumsiness	√				√			
Tremors/Shakes	√				√			
Thoughts of Suicide	√				√			
Agoraphobia	√				√			
Increased Physical Activity	√				√			
Heavy/Aching Legs	√				√			
Generalized Aches	√				√			
Bad Breath	√				√			
Sensitivity to Music/Light	√				√			
Excessive Thirst	√				√			

and have a bowl of bran. I also drank about five cups of tea per day, an extra ¾ of a pint (450 ml) of milk per day, and other dairy foods.

On my programme I was asked to cut out grains, dairy products, yeast-based foods, tea and foods containing sugar. I stuck to the diet to the letter. It was inconvenient at first because it was so different. It took me a week or two to adapt and then it became easier.

Miraculously, soon after I began the diet my tummy problems just cleared up. I now know through trial and error that wheat and dairy products are irritants and will cause my diarrhoea to return.

I have relaxed my diet now that I am so much better. I am still fairly strict with myself most of the time. I can get away with drinking alcohol occasionally and sometimes I do eat processed foods or crisps.

End result

Now that I have followed the nutritional programme, I have learned so much. My body has recovered from all the ailments, including my PMS and the irritable bowel syndrome. All the remaining traces of agoraphobia which I had previously suffered from in my late teens and early twenties have disappeared, and my skin condition has improved. My energy has just soared and I feel that I have come from being a poorly, lethargic person suddenly to someone who is healthy all the time. I am my usual bouncy self once again and I get on well with people. I don't experience the miseries any more, I am relieved to say.

I honestly feel that the Women's Nutritional Advisory Service has transformed my life. I used to think life was terrible. Now I find life pleasurable. I feel healthier than I have ever done, at least since I was a child. I can't thank them enough.'

Nadine had no symptoms whatsoever left at the end of her six-month programme, as you can see from her chart.

An extract from a letter explains how Nadine felt about her programme.

'I wanted to make some additional comments regarding the programme, apart from those in the accompanying questionnaire.

First of all, I'd like to thank you for such detailed information and guidance in your letter of recommendations. The programme has made the biological and physiological aspects of womanhood a great deal easier to cope with. My periods are much less painful and lighter. The gruesome week before my period, which was always so unbearable, is now like the other two weeks. I no longer suffer from any breast tenderness, which used to be so severe, and no longer suffer with bloatedness. I no longer hate everything and everybody including myself, and I no longer feel violent or aggressive, which is a very great relief. I also don't wreck everything around me through clumsiness, as that's gone too.

All in all, the programme has transformed me and my life quite remarkably and I am grateful for the work you and your colleagues have done to enable me to live without dreading the onset of each period. More significantly, I feel that the diet and discovery of foods that I am allergic to has improved my whole life, not just my PMS.

For about seven years I have suffered with irritable bowel syndrome, more recently it became so bad that I was referred to a specialist who, after various unpleasant tests, pronounced it was caused by stress. Ironically most doctors have prescribed increased intake of wholewheat products and bran, no wonder I wasn't getting any better! Admittedly, when I am in a stressful situation my symptoms return, but they last only as long as the stress. Previously, the irritable bowel symptoms were with me constantly and just became unbearable when I was under stress.

I know this isn't entirely relevant to your work on PMS but at the same time many of my female contemporaries seem to suffer from irritable bowel syndrome too and I wonder how many women are being inappropriately treated and dismissed with mutterings of ''it's psychosomatic''?

I hope my comments have been some help in your work to relieve the misery of PMS. I for one am a very grateful and satisfied customer!'

Yours sincerely
Nadine

6

BLOATING, WEIGHT GAIN AND BREAST TENDERNESS

PMS H (HYDRATION)

PMS H sufferers complain of weight gain pre-menstrually. The hands and feet often swell so that rings and shoes become too tight. The face often becomes puffy and the waistline expands so that clothes feel too tight. The abdomen can become bloated and tender and the same applies to the breasts.

The manifestations of these symptoms are mostly physical, in that women report feeling very uncomfortable and often sore. Because of their increased size many women feel self-conscious and get very touchy and introverted. Surprisingly, most women who suffer from PMS H only gain up to 3–4 pounds (1–2 kg) pre-menstrually. Approximately 20 per cent seem to gain far more than this. I have personally seen women who gain up to 12 pounds (5.4 kg) before their periods. They literally change dress size and need to have two sets of underwear to cope with their increased breast size.

Symptoms due to excess fluid retention can easily be worsened by eating the wrong diet. A high intake of sodium or ordinary salt, which is the norm in the United Kingdom, is the commonest cause of fluid retention in women. It appears that some women are particularly prone to develop fluid retention whereas others can eat salty foods with impunity. Thus part of the programme for those with fluid retention symptoms is to greatly reduce the intake of salt from that used in the cooking, that added to food at the table and from salty foods. Nowadays, like our consumption of sugar, at least two-thirds of the salt we eat is 'hidden' in common foods such as bacon, ham, sausages, other preserved meat products, cheeses, most butters and margarines, bread, tinned foods like tinned tuna and vegetables, salted crisps and nuts and most savoury snacks and convenience meals.

Good old plain fruit and vegetables, meat, fish, beans and rice are all low in sodium and have good levels of potassium. A good intake of potassium and magnesium from the diet may help minimize the effects of too much sodium. Fortunately there are many low-salt (sodium) versions of tinned and other foods now available.

Consuming a lot of carbohydrate-rich foods and sugar, including that from soft drinks, which many women drink in substantial quantities premenstrually, can also lead to fluid retention. Curiously, drinking a lot of water, low-calorie drinks and even tea and coffee without sugar does not cause this problem. Losing weight if you are overweight may also help with fluid retention symptoms.

However, some women who complain of pre-menstrual abdominal bloating and puffy fingers do not have an increase in body water and salt content. It may be that their perception of their body changes and they just 'feel' different.

THE DEGREE OF SUFFERING

In our survey we found that 90.8 per cent of the women complained of abdominal bloating to some degree, (72 per cent severe to moderately).

Of the women studied 86.8 per cent had pre-menstrual breast tenderness (67 per cent severe to moderate sufferers).

Weight was gained by 84 per cent (52 per cent severe to moderately) and 54 per cent complained of swelling of the extremities (33 per cent severe to moderate).

Degree of pre-menstrual breast tenderness suffered out of a sample of 1000 women

Not Affected	Mild	Moderate	Severe	Total Affected
13.2%	19.9%	31.6%	35.3%	- 86.8%

Degree to which abdominal bloating affected a sample of 1000 women pre-menstrually

Not Affected	Mild	Moderate	Severe	Total Affected
9.2%	18.5%	39.3%	33.0%	- 90.8%

WEIGHT LOSS

Whilst conducting our follow-up consultations during the programme and in our clinics, we began to notice that many overweight women who were previously unable to lose weight were enthusiastically reporting weight loss. This began occurring even after the first month, without even 'dieting' to lose weight. In fact, their intake of food during the programme was in many cases greater than usual.

Because of this somewhat unexpected outcome, we decided to monitor a group of 50 PMS sufferers who were also overweight, through the first three months of their programme. (Thirty-six of the women were at least 10 per cent overweight and 14 of them were obese, which means greater than 33 per cent above normal body weight.) The symptoms complained of most severely to begin with were weight gain, fatigue, abdominal bloating, craving for food, in particular sweet foods, and anxiety.

After three months on their programmes there was an 84 per cent reduction in severe symptoms.

The overweight group of 36 women lost an average of 7 pounds (3 kg) and the obese group of 14 women lost an average of 13 pounds (6 kg) in this three-month period.

We can't say precisely why this amount of weight loss had occurred, particularly when the women had previously found it difficult to lose weight. However, the common denominator seems to be that they were all on a healthy diet that had been balanced according to their individual needs. We therefore suspect that this must have had a positive effect on their metabolism with the result that they began to shed excess weight.

This is certainly an area we would like to research further. But in the meantime it's a gift horse that won't be looked in the mouth by PMS H sufferers.

" Dee's Story "

Dee is a full-time mother of two from Dunstable in Bedfordshire.

'Whenever I was invited out I had to check my diary twice, once to see whether I was free and the other to see how near to my period it was. If the date was anything up to 16 days before my period I knew that I would be so bloated I wouldn't be able to fit into any of my usual clothes. I had one outfit that fitted pre-menstrually and that was it. My husband would ask about my new dress or skirt that I had bought only days before, and I'd have to admit that it didn't fit now. I am usually a size 12, but pre-menstrually I gained four inches around my waist. I also suffered with

headaches, insomnia, continual tiredness and sore throats, and found it very difficult to cope.

I actually didn't realize that I was suffering with PMS until I read a feature on the Women's Nutritional Advisory Service. The article listed all my symptoms. All at once I felt I had a reason for feeling as I did.

Diet reduced my bloating

I contacted the WNAS and followed their postal programme. They thought the fluid retention was related to my salt and caffeine intake. I had previously been snacking on crisps and drinking lots of strong tea. I followed the programme written for me, and had my monthly consultations during the programme. I noticed a real improvement within ten days, and within three months my symptoms had disappeared. At last I feel I'm in control of my body. It's a pain not to eat everything I'd like, but feeling good all month is easily worth that – and I only need one wardrobe of clothes.

〈〈 Rebecca's Story 〉〉

Rebecca is a 38-year-old divorcee with two children who works as a teacher.

'Looking back, I think my symptoms began increasing in severity after the birth of my children. Certainly, the last ten years have been the worst. I suffered for years before I even knew what I was suffering from. I'd never heard of "PMS". My doctor was unsympathetic, and so I thought it was just part of my make-up and therefore something I had to suffer.

My husband was very unsympathetic towards me during my premenstrual times. He couldn't believe I could be all right one minute and then suddenly have symptoms which involved him making adjustments. He really doubted that my symptoms actually existed. It caused a lot of misunderstandings and arguments. For example, I remember a time when I asked him to turn the record player down as it was giving me a headache, and he just grudgingly said, "Well, you were quite all right this morning". I just used to feel depressed, isolated and confused because I didn't really know why I was feeling so different pre-menstrually.

44

My symptoms would occur 10 to 12 days pre-menstrually. The most physically noticeable thing was that I'd gain four to five pounds (2–3 kg) in weight; my abdomen felt really bloated. I'd get cravings for food, in fact I just couldn't seem to get satisfied no matter what I ate. Apart from that I'd feel very irritable, exhausted and fairly afraid of my dizziness and fainting attacks, particularly when I went shopping or stood up for any length of time.

I looked terrible pre-menstrually, which didn't help. I had puffy eyes surrounded by dark shadows. Another thing was that I used to always feel cold, an inner cold. I would have to go to bed and crawl under the duvet with a hot-water bottle, but still wouldn't be able to overcome the cold; my teeth would still be chattering.

Life was really very difficult at the time and the stress of a broken marriage made things even worse. I found it difficult to work pre-menstrually as I couldn't concentrate. My head was so fuzzy and I couldn't formulate my ideas properly.

I had previously tried several different treatments for PMS, none of which were of any lasting value. I tried taking vitamin B6 on its own, but it didn't work. I also had some acupuncture and visited a medical herbalist. I put myself on to a course of Efamol evening primrose oil, but found that this only helped initially.

Scatterbrain!

I was so forgetful. One day I put my handbag on the roof of the car whilst I loaded it and then I drove off without moving it! I can honestly say I felt terrible pre-menstrually. I didn't like myself at all.

Wrecked marriage

My marriage broke down. I know that my PMS symptoms aggravated the situation. They caused a lot of misunderstandings. We had awful rows. He simply didn't believe my symptoms existed. I think he thought I'd made them up to suit myself and to inconvenience him. He had no understanding of the situation and I felt so isolated in it. I got very confused and tense as a result which aggravated my behaviour, so it was a vicious circle.'

Rebecca had severe symptoms in all four categories, pre-menstrually, whereas she had practically no symptoms at all at any other time of the month.

Rebecca also had 'before' and 'after' laboratory tests during her treatment which are detailed on page 138.

'When I heard about the nutritional approach to PMS, I decided to give it a go. I have been under Dr Stewart for over a year now. He has been measuring levels of vitamins and minerals in my body. I discovered I had an added complication of severe food allergies which we have also been working on, and a thyroid problem which is now being treated. My symptoms are down to a bearable two days per month now and I hope that I will be able to overcome them completely as time goes on.

Robert, with whom I now live, is very understanding and tolerant. Whenever I couldn't cope with a situation, he would just help me to do something. I'm sure it's due to his support that I have made it through.'

7

SUGAR CRAVINGS, HEADACHES AND FATIGUE

PMS C (CARBOHYDRATE CRAVING)

In this sub-group of PMS, one to two weeks before the period the appetite increases. Cravings for food begin, particularly for sweet foods and chocolate. Often stress intensifies the situation. Satisfying the cravings is a vicious circle. A typical example is as follows.

The day starts with either no breakfast or just a couple of cups of tea or coffee and a few cigarettes. This may stimulate the body's metabolism and one's energy for a short while, but the problems begin by mid-morning. By this time the energy level tends to fall, and symptoms of nervousness, anxiety, palpitations, light headaches, hunger and cravings for food, particularly sweet foods, set in. Another cup of tea or coffee with sugar, or with a sugary or chocolate snack, may delay symptoms for a while but nothing short of a good wholesome meal will resolve these symptoms.

Some of these symptoms may be due to a fall in the level of sugar (glucose) in the blood – known as hypoglycaemia. As the brain and nervous system rely upon glucose for their source of energy, a fall in its level can cause a whole host of nervous system symptoms. The body compensates by producing adrenaline, which increases the level of glucose in the blood, but aggravates symptoms of anxiety, palpitations, sweating and shaking.

Such symptoms may be improved by the next meal. Often the mid-morning or mid-afternoon fatigue or sweet cravings are relieved by a wholesome lunch, supper or snack.

Not all women will have such marked symptoms, nor indeed will there always be marked swings in blood sugar levels. Often one just feels better if one eats three good meals a day, a couple of healthy snacks, and has a regular, not too hectic lifestyle.

Headaches can also be caused by excessive intake of tea and coffee. Fatigue can be affected by the balance of minerals, such as iron and magnesium. Any women with persistent fatigue should certainly see her doctor for examination and appropriate blood tests, particularly to check for anaemia or reduced activity of the thyroid gland.

GOOD FOOD REGULARLY, PLEASE!

So often the cravings for sweet foods, sugary snacks and chocolate are the result of an irregular and inadequate diet. Women with PMS C – carbo-hydrate cravings – may also experience headache, increased appetite, heart pounding, fatigue, and dizziness and fainting. These symptoms can be due to the swings in blood sugar levels and over-reliance on social stimulants: caffeine from tea, coffee, cola, chocolate, alcohol, cigarettes and even marijuana. Three good, regular meals, two wholesome in-be-tween-meal snacks and cutting down on sugar and social stimulants are all essential to treat PMS C.

THE DEGREE OF SUFFERING

In our study we found that 77 per cent of the women were suffering with cravings for sweet food, just over 60 per cent severe to moderately. There were 93 per cent who reported suffering with fatigue pre-menstrually, 82 per cent severe to moderately; 77 per cent reported headaches pre-menstrually, 74 per cent general increased appetite, 53 per cent heart pounding and 50 per cent dizziness and fainting.

" Geraldine's Story "

Geraldine is a 33-year-old mother of three who works as a nursing auxili-ary. She had had PMS since 1983, after the birth of her third baby.

She had severe symptoms in all four categories. She felt 'possessed' pre-menstrually and hardly recognized herself. She was withdrawn from life and disgusted with her own behaviour. Her eating habits were particularly erratic pre-menstrually. In particular she craved chocolate, which she felt immensely guilty about.

'I thought sometimes I could just sit zombie-like and not talk to anybody. I wanted to go to the doctor and ask him to take my children and put me in a white jacket and stick me in a room somewhere. In fact, it even makes me feel bad talking about it.

Post-natal depression

When my third child was three months old I suddenly developed post-natal depression. It hit me really hard as I had never experienced it before. I didn't feel aggressive towards the baby, I just knew there was something wrong with me. I used to sit staring into space for hours. There were jobs that needed doing and the whole house was disintegrating, but I just couldn't do anything. I felt awful all the time and I had no energy or enthusiasm. I was overweight and depressed.

My doctor prescribed anti-depressants. I don't know if they helped or not. They helped me to sleep, but I was afraid I wouldn't wake up. They made me feel zombie-like.

I realized I had PMS during a sticky patch in my marriage. I felt I was reacting to everything and that some problem had to be present in order to make me feel so bad.

49

Black cloud overhead

Whereas I hadn't felt aggressive with post-natal depression, I felt absolutely horrendous when I had PMS. I used to feel I had an individual black cloud hanging over me. I'd wake up in the morning knowing that awful feeling was there and that there was nothing I could do to make it go away. I just knew I had days ahead of me feeling so awful.

I didn't want to participate in my usual activities pre-menstrually. I belong to an amateur dramatics society, but I just didn't feel I could do anything like that. You need to give a lot of yourself in things like that, and I didn't feel capable of doing what I was supposed to do. My memory just went, and I would literally go blank, and that applied to everything, not just my drama.

I felt like a zombie and wanted to withdraw from life. I was disgusted with my behaviour towards the children, who, as a result, are quite afraid of me. To compensate I'd then eat vast quantities of chocolate for comfort which would only serve to make my symptoms worse.

I often found myself hiding away to eat in private. I found the amount I was eating an embarrassment. If you fancy a bar of chocolate you go off and buy one and that's fine. But I could eat four or five bars at once, and then eat the same amount again. You can't get rid of that many sweet papers. So you gradually ease them out of your pocket, or wrap them in something else, and throw them in the bin. The children would notice I'd had more than one bar; I couldn't pull the wool over their eyes. I wasn't aware that I was being silly at the time, I just used to sit and eat and then feel so sick afterwards.

I knew I wouldn't do any housework in the days to come, and that I wouldn't want to do anything with the children. I would be unbearable to my husband and I wouldn't bother to cook.

My doctor again prescribed anti-depressants. But knowing they made me feel zombie-like, I didn't want to take them any more. I was also prescribed diuretics. Unfortunately they seem to stop my bladder working properly, because I can't make it to the loo in time. So they were really out anyway.

I also tried vitamin B6, evening primrose oil, multi-vitamins, ginseng and progesterone pessaries.

At the time I felt life wasn't really worth living. I existed from situation to situation. It was a very stressful time. I had one good week in four. It was unbearable for the family; it was really horrible. I thought I was going round the bend, totally insane and that no one could help me at all. I didn't really know who to contact as I'd tried all my doctor had to offer. I then read an article in a women's magazine about the nutritional approach to PMS and the work the Stewarts were doing.'

PRE-MENSTRUAL SYNDROME QUESTIONNAIRE

Name: Geraldine Ellis   Age: 32   Height: 5' 9"   Weight: 10st 7lb

MARITAL STATUS: Single _____   Married _✓_   Divorced _____   Widowed _____
(Please tick where applicable)

PRESENT CONTRACEPTION: None _____   Pill _____   I.U.D. _____   Other _✓_

Your periods come every __28__ days   Your periods last _7–8_ days

Your periods are: Light _____   Moderate _✓_   Heavy _____

Number of Pregnancies: __3__   Number of Miscarriages: _____

Birth weight of children:
1st child _7lb 3oz_   2nd child _8lb 1oz_   3rd child _8lb 11oz_   4th child _____

SYMPTOMS	WEEK AFTER PERIOD (Fill in 3 days after period)				WEEK BEFORE PERIOD (Fill in 2-3 days before period)			
	None	Mild	Moderate	Severe	None	Mild	Moderate	Severe
PMS - A								
Nervous Tension	✓					✓		
Mood Swings	✓						✓	
Irritability	✓							✓
Anxiety	✓				✓			
PMS - H								
Weight Gain	✓						✓	
Swelling of Extremities	✓							✓
Breast Tenderness	✓					✓		
Abdominal Bloating	✓						✓	
PMS - C								
Headache	✓						✓	
Craving for Sweets	✓							✓
Increased Appetite	✓							✓
Heart Pounding	✓				✓			
Fatigue	✓							✓
Dizziness or Fainting	✓				✓			
PMS - D								
Depression	✓							✓
Forgetfulness	✓						✓	
Crying	✓							✓
Confusion	✓						✓	
Insomnia	✓						✓	
OTHER SYMPTOMS								
Loss of Sexual Interest	✓							✓
Disorientation	✓				✓			
Clumsiness	✓						✓	
Tremors/Shakes	✓				✓			
Thoughts of Suicide	✓					✓		
Agoraphobia	✓							✓
Increased Physical Activity	✓				✓			
Heavy/Aching Legs	✓						✓	
Generalized Aches	✓					✓		
Bad Breath	✓				✓			
Sensitivity to Music/Light	✓				✓			
Excessive Thirst	✓				✓			

FOLLOW UP
PRE-MENSTRUAL SYNDROME QUESTIONNAIRE

Name: Geraldine Ellis   Age: 32   Height: 5' 9"   Weight: 10st

MARITAL STATUS: Single _____ Married __√__ Divorced _____ Widowed _____
(Please tick where applicable)

PRESENT CONTRACEPTION: None_____ Pill_____ I.U.D._____ Other __√__

Your periods come every __28__ days   Your periods last __7–8__ days

Your periods are: Light_____ Moderate___√___ Heavy_____

SYMPTOMS

	WEEK AFTER PERIOD (Fill in 3 days after period)				WEEK BEFORE PERIOD (Fill in 2-3 days before period)			
	None	Mild	Moderate	Severe	None	Mild	Moderate	Severe
PMS - A								
Nervous Tension	√				√			
Mood Swings	√				√			
Irritability	√				√			
Anxiety	√				√			
PMS - H								
Weight Gain	√						√	
Swelling of Extremities	√				√			
Breast Tenderness	√				√			
Abdominal Bloating	√						√	
PMS - C								
Headache	√				√			
Craving for Sweets	√						√	
Increased Appetite	√				√			
Heart Pounding	√				√			
Fatigue	√				√			
Dizziness or Fainting	√				√			
PMS - D								
Depression	√				√			
Forgetfulness	√				√			
Crying	√				√			
Confusion	√				√			
Insomnia	√				√			
OTHER SYMPTOMS								
Loss of Sexual Interest	√				√			
Disorientation	√				√			
Clumsiness	√				√			
Tremors/Shakes	√				√			
Thoughts of Suicide	√				√			
Agoraphobia	√				√			
Increased Physical Activity	√				√			
Heavy/Aching Legs	√				√			
Generalized Aches	√				√			
Bad Breath	√				√			
Sensitivity to Music/Light	√				√			
Excessive Thirst	√				√			

One of Geraldine's particular weaknesses was her craving for sweet food pre-menstrually and her excessive indulgence. Later on in Chapter 11, I will be talking about the detrimental effects of excessive amounts of sweet food, particularly in relation to PMS symptoms.

On her first chart Geraldine's worst symptoms were in the sub-groups PMS C and PMS D, although she did have severe symptoms in all four categories.

Like the majority of women, Geraldine was lacking in education about the importance of a correct diet. This is hardly surprising considering how little we learned at school about nutrition as a subject. Until recent times very little attention has been placed on the role of nutrition in relation to women's health.

> 'I knew a bit about diet, but had no idea that changing my diet could bring me back to normal, and that's what it has done. Although I didn't know that I was sensitive to any foods, I had a good idea what was and what wasn't a sensible diet. My trouble was temptation. It's much easier to buy chocolate, which is available wherever you go, than it is to go home and make fish cakes with sesame seeds on them or things like that which you know are much better for you. I did eat healthy things, but I also ate a load of rubbish.
>
> I try to stick to the diet. I feel much better when I do. I know I shouldn't eat chocolates, processed food, salty food or wheat. I did try some Stilton cheese and crisps, but I blew up like a balloon shortly after eating them. I now know that chocolate makes me depressed and, of course, I put on weight if I eat rubbish.

End result

> Since I've been following the nutritional programme I feel so much better. My children notice the difference in me; I am no longer nasty to them. It has made me feel so much better in myself. I personally feel fine, although I could still do with losing weight.
>
> I still have my marital problems. But I know that we have got things wrong marriage-wise, I know they are not related to PMS. I haven't got that aggressiveness inside me so much and I haven't got that awful feeling, that black cloud hanging over my head. That was the worst thing.'

Geraldine's follow-up chart verifies her story. Apart from a few remaining mild symptoms at the time of writing, she felt that she had overcome her PMS.

Another victim of chocolate cravings was Anita Walker. Her addiction to chocolate was no secret. It ran her life. She admits that she had little control over it. When you read her story, she could so easily be talking about a drug or alcohol.

ANITA WALKER – SUGAR CRAVINGS

'I am actually embarrassed to tell you about my sugar cravings. I would eat masses of chocolate bars, I could eat two bags of fun-size chocolate bars, or seven or eight ordinary bars and half a cake, and then eat my tea.

The more I ate, the worse my cravings would be, it was a vicious circle. I would feel OK for a bit after eating all that, and then I would feel awful. Especially more irritable, and especially more aggressive!

I didn't recognize that this was happening pre-menstrually at the time. I felt as though the toxins were building up and I would have to go to bed early, feeling fat and sick and having eaten myself into a stupor.'

I'm hardly surprised that Anita felt embarrassed to relate this part of her story. She was a real 'chocoholic'. Fortunately, we were able to relieve her of these cravings early on in her programme. Over the years we have had great success treating cravings for sweet food. If this is your main problem you may be interested to read about the latest research and how to overcome the problems in the book *Beat Sugar Craving*. See page 251 for details. In the Self-Help section on page 182 I will explain how Anita also managed to overcome her thrush.

8

DEPRESSION, CRYING AND THOUGHTS OF SUICIDE

PMS D (DEPRESSION)

Depression is a common pre-menstrual symptom and usually is present with other symptoms such as anxiety and breast tenderness. Our own research has shown that those most likely to suffer from pre-menstrual depression are more often overweight and do less exercise than those who do not suffer so badly with this problem.

The balance of certain nutrients has an important influence on both hormone and brain chemistry. Magnesium, for example, influences how the ovaries respond in the normal menstrual cycles, and many other nutrients are also important in this respect. It is also known that in people with severe depression the chance of finding some degree of B vitamin deficiency is much higher than would be expected in the general population. These nutrients have been used successfully in treating both PMS and depression.

In our study we found that 94 per cent of the women suffered from pre-menstrual depression, 83.8 per cent severe to moderately. This, we felt, was a frighteningly high number, and in view of the possible consequences of depression, not something that should be taken lightly.

Degree to which 1000 women suffered depression pre-menstrually				
Not Affected	Mild	Moderate	Severe	Total Affected
6%	10.2%	29.9%	53.9% -	94%

In 1959 Dr Katharina Dalton published a study in the *British Medical Journal* which showed that the time of admission to hospital of depressed patients coincided with the menstrual period, the pre-menstrual phase, and ovulation.

The balance of hormones – or whatever determines their balance, seems to be crucial in controlling mood. We are beginning to learn how diet and lifestyle can influence our hormones and our moods.

Time of admission of 185 patients with depression.
(From Dalton K. (1959). Br. Med. J.; 1:148–149.)

SUICIDAL

Many women who were suffering with PMS D reported that they felt suicidal, indeed it was because we were coming across so many women who felt suicidal that we decided to embark on the study of 1000 women.

Tragically, we found that 41 per cent of them had previously contemplated suicide pre-menstrually, 35 per cent of them several times and 5.8 per cent had actually attempted suicide pre-menstrually. That is a staggering 58 women out of 1000 that were chosen.

Suicidal tendencies out of a sample of 1000 women

Once	More than once	More than six times	Total	Attempted
6.0%	23.3%	12.1%	41.4%	5.8%

A group of French doctors have linked attempted suicide in the pre-menstrual phase with low levels of the hormone oestrogen. However, some of the women had normal or even high levels of this hormone. For some an imbalance in this hormone might affect brain chemistry and thus mood. A healthy diet, exercise, nutritional supplements and controlling stress are the types of approaches that can help normalize hormone and body chemistry and thus decrease pre-menstrual depression.

Time of acute psychiatric admission in 276 patients.
(From Dalton K. (1959). Br. Med. J.; 1:148–149.)

Again in 1959 Dr Dalton looked at the timing of 276 acute psychiatric admissions in four London hospitals. According to her findings, which were published in the *British Medical Journal*, 46 per cent of the patients were admitted between the 25th day of their cycle and the 4th day of their new cycle.

Also 53 per cent of attempted suicides, 47 per cent of admissions for depression and 47 per cent of schizophrenic patients were admitted during these eight days of the menstrual cycle.

" Sally's Story "

Sally is a 38-year-old woman who works as a recruitment consultant. She was married previously, but is now divorced.

Sally seriously contemplated taking a whole bottle of pills when she was pre-menstrual. Fortunately, she saw the light in time and relates the story to us as if she were talking about someone else.

'I really thought I was mentally ill, mentally inadequate; I thought I was cracking up. I was frightened to tell people how I felt because they might have thought I was a loony.

I did seriously contemplate suicide once. It was a bad time for me anyway as I was under a lot of stress. Being pre-menstrual was the last straw and I did contemplate taking a whole bottle of pills. Fortunately, I have some faith in God and I'm sure that's what eventually pulled me together and stopped me.

I felt that I was unbalanced and I couldn't stand the pain that the depression inside was causing any more. I just wanted to go to sleep so that it would all end.

PMS meant the pain of depression. I felt absolute despair pre-menstrually and I cannot express in words how desolate this made me feel. I really thought I was mentally ill. I thought my mind was taking over. Anything and everything was too stressful for me, and I felt I just couldn't cope.

Stress
I would say stress definitely did influence my symptoms. When I was under stress I tended to get a runny tummy, therefore I don't suppose I

got the full benefit of my food. It's like a vicious circle to me. When I'm under stress I don't eat, and then as a result I feel even more stressed.

However, since I have been following the programme I am definitely less affected by stress. I seem much more able to cope with stressful situations, which I certainly wouldn't have been able to cope with before.

I tried vitamin B6. It wasn't any help, but I think I know why. I discovered on the programme that I have a sensitivity to yeast, and the B6 tablets I was taking were yeast-based. I found that the B6 would perk me up and then I would drop down mentally and have a terrible bloated tummy.

I also tried evening primrose oil, which helped with the breast symptoms. I was prescribed anti-depressants, which were no help at all. They just made me feel out of control. They controlled a bit of the depression, but they just made me void of other emotions.

I didn't really recognize my symptoms as PMS. That was the worst thing, looking back. I just knew I was suffering with depression and agoraphobia regularly, in fact towards the end, most of the time. I only had one good week after my period, the rest of the time was distressing. When I first saw the Women's Nutritional Advisory Service questionnaire and realized that agoraphobic symptoms could be part of the Pre-Menstrual Syndrome it gave me a great sense of relief. I felt a bit better just knowing that my symptoms were part of PMS. It gave me a far greater understanding of my suffering.

I thought I would give the nutritional approach to PMS a try as I felt so unwell, and I was so sick of taking anti-depressants and sleeping tablets. I had to do something as I honestly felt I was cracking up.'

Imagine having to live with the secret that you thought you were mentally ill. As a divorcee, Sally had to fend for herself.

Her job and her income were exceedingly important and she obviously thought these were threatened by her severe symptoms. She had tried several solutions, like our other patients, but did not find her symptoms lessened.

She suffered pre-menstrually with severe symptoms in all four categories, as her chart shows. She also had pre-menstrual agoraphobia, which was a terrific handicap in her working and social life.

The power of diet

'I used to eat lots of bread, cakes, animal fats including lots of butter and drink a substantial amount of tea and coffee.

PRE-MENSTRUAL SYNDROME QUESTIONNAIRE

Name: Sally Noone   Age: 38   Height: 5' 3"   Weight: 9st

MARITAL STATUS: Single _____   Married _____   Divorced √   Widowed _____
(Please tick where applicable)

PRESENT CONTRACEPTION: None_____   Pill_____   I.U.D._____   Other √

Your periods come every   29   days   Your periods last   3   days

Your periods are: Light_____   Moderate √   Heavy_____

Number of Pregnancies: –   Number of Miscarriages: –

Birth weight of children:
1st child_____   2nd child_____   3rd child_____   4th child_____

SYMPTOMS	WEEK AFTER PERIOD (Fill in 3 days after period)				WEEK BEFORE PERIOD (Fill in 2-3 days before period)			
	None	Mild	Moderate	Severe	None	Mild	Moderate	Severe
PMS - A								
Nervous Tension			√					√
Mood Swings			√					√
Irritability			√					√
Anxiety			√					√
PMS - H								
Weight Gain	√							√
Swelling of Extremities	√					√		
Breast Tenderness	√						√	
Abdominal Bloating		√						√
PMS - C								
Headache		√				√		
Craving for Sweets	√							√
Increased Appetite	√							√
Heart Pounding		√						√
Fatigue			√					√
Dizziness or Fainting	√							√
PMS - D								
Depression		√						√
Forgetfulness		√						√
Crying			√					√
Confusion		√						√
Insomnia		√						√
OTHER SYMPTOMS								
Loss of Sexual Interest				√				√
Disorientation		√						√
Clumsiness		√					√	
Tremors/Shakes	√							√
Thoughts of Suicide	√							√
Agoraphobia	√							√
Increased Physical Activity	√							√
Heavy/Aching Legs		√				√		
Generalized Aches		√					√	
Bad Breath	√							√
Sensitivity to Music/Light	√							√
Excessive Thirst	√							√

FOLLOW UP
PRE-MENSTRUAL SYNDROME QUESTIONNAIRE

Name: Sally Noone   Age: 38   Height: 5' 3"   Weight: 8st 9lb

MARITAL STATUS: Single ✓ Married _____ Divorced _____ Widowed _____
(Please tick where applicable)

PRESENT CONTRACEPTION: None ✓ Pill _____ I.U.D. _____ Other _____

    Your periods come every __28__ days   Your periods last __3__ days

    Your periods are: Light _____ Moderate __✓__ Heavy _____

SYMPTOMS

Symptom	WEEK AFTER PERIOD (Fill in 3 days after period)				WEEK BEFORE PERIOD (Fill in 2-3 days before period)			
	None	Mild	Moderate	Severe	None	Mild	Moderate	Severe
PMS - A								
Nervous Tension	✓					✓		
Mood Swings	✓				✓			
Irritability	✓					✓		
Anxiety	✓					✓		
PMS - H								
Weight Gain	✓				✓			
Swelling of Extremities	✓				✓			
Breast Tenderness	✓					✓		
Abdominal Bloating	✓				✓			
PMS - C								
Headache	✓				✓			
Craving for Sweets	✓					✓		
Increased Appetite	✓				✓			
Heart Pounding	✓				✓			
Fatigue	✓				✓			
Dizziness or Fainting	✓				✓			
PMS - D								
Depression	✓					✓		
Forgetfulness	✓				✓			
Crying	✓				✓			
Confusion	✓				✓			
Insomnia	✓				✓			
OTHER SYMPTOMS								
Loss of Sexual Interest		✓			✓			
Disorientation	✓				✓			
Clumsiness	✓					✓		
Tremors/Shakes	✓				✓			
Thoughts of Suicide	✓				✓			
Agoraphobia	✓				✓			
Increased Physical Activity	✓				✓			
Heavy/Aching Legs	✓				✓			
Generalized Aches	✓				✓			
Bad Breath	✓				✓			
Sensitivity to Music/Light	✓				✓			
Excessive Thirst	✓				✓			

I had no idea that my symptoms could be diet-related until I read an article in a magazine. I realized at that point that it was likely that something in my diet might be making me feel so bad.

The diet recommended was a bit bewildering at first, probably because it's so different. I was asked to come off grains for a short period, and to omit all foods with a yeast base from my diet. I had to cut down my junk food intake, including sugary foods, i.e. biscuits, cakes, puddings. Also to cut down on salt, alcohol and dairy products.

There are many alternative foods to eat and I soon got used to the diet. In fact I feel I have now revamped my whole way of eating, and I enjoy my food more. I found that I have a sensitivity to wheat, sugar and chocolate. If I eat them I get a reaction the next day. I get a mild sort of dizziness and windy stomach. I know now that it is going to be over within 24 hours, whereas before I would get so upset and confused because I wouldn't know what was causing it. To tell the truth, when my tummy used to swell, I really thought I had cancer.

My symptoms disappeared on the programme. The depression cleared within one week and the remaining symptoms gradually disappeared during the first three months. So much so, I decided I no longer needed to follow the recommendations. Coming off the diet and reverting to my previous diet brought the symptoms back. I went back on to the programme recommended, and within a short space of time my symptoms were under control again. I've proved to myself that the diet works for me.

I have been taking Optivite since I started the programme. That, the exercise and the diet have done so much good for me. I really think that Optivite is the best thing since sliced bread.

End result

Now that I have been through the programme, I am much more stable. I am able to stick at my job and maintain my concentration. I have a very stressful job, but I am now able to work hard and I feel very happy. PMS does not affect me any more. The programme has changed my life. I can cope better with everything. I would say I am a thousand times better. I no longer feel exhausted after little effort. I am so delighted. Looking back, it's like looking at a different person.'

Once again you can see that Sally's symptoms have gone from severe to mild in just a few months. She feels her life has returned to normal because she followed the nutritional programme, which is reflected in her final chart and letter as follows.

Dear Maryon,

I am writing to let you know that there is a marked change in my life. I feel that I have come through the proverbial 'long dark tunnel' out of despair into sunlight. If only I had known about the yeast allergy years ago and trusted my instinct about magnesium, the before and after picture shown on the symptom tables would not have been so acutely marked!

I think because I had hidden all the symptoms and bottled them up, my family are not really aware of the change I feel inside. There was certainly scepticism from one branch of my family when I tried to explain it to them, and why I was being 'faddish' about my food. The knowledge that certain foods will send me back into the downward spiral of depression is enough to ensure that I steer clear of any of them, and keep to the new regime.

I am getting to be a bore with some of my friends. As soon as they start complaining about any of the symptoms I used to have, I try to analyse their diet for them and I also give them your address – whether they want it or not!

I do hope you manage to get the message across to all the women who need it – for anyone else to suffer the way I did, and not to know the way out – well, it is criminal and so much more must be done.

Sally Noone
(a convert)

PMS D can be very severe indeed. We have dealt with some very sad cases, where women felt suicidal, depressed and that life was not worth living pre-menstrually.

The first example I will give you is the story of Anita Walker.

" Anita's Story "

Anita is a 36-year-old mother of two children who works as a personnel assistant. Her PMS began when she was 17 years old, but became worse about eight years ago after having children and a miscarriage. She has also had a hysterectomy due to excessive bleeding and fibroids.

'I ended up with only four or five normal days per month. The rest of the time, apart from my period, I'd get fatter and fatter. I'd feel tired and

irritable and couldn't concentrate, to the point where I didn't know what day of the week it was.

I attacked my husband with a knife on several occasions. I kept away from the baby as I was terrified of baby battering; I knew I could so easily have done it.

I remember feeling suicidal and not knowing where I was. I'd find myself out in the street yelling in the middle of the night, this happened pre-menstrually. It was like being Jekyll and Hyde. I'd be totally irrational and make stupid decisions. The week after, I'd look back and wonder why on earth I acted that way.

One night, a week before my period, feeling nobody cared, I thought I just couldn't go on any more. I felt fat, depressed and I didn't think life was worth living for a week to ten days before my period. I was utterly desperate. I got this bottle of wine and my nice collection of sleeping pills that my doctor had doled out. I just quietly swallowed the lot, and the next thing I knew I was waking up in hospital, wondering what I was doing there.

No connection was made there between my condition and PMS. They just told me to go away, not to be a silly girl, and to stop upsetting my family. No treatment offered by my doctor made any lasting impact on my symptoms.

What about me?

I never liked myself pre-menstrually. I really did feel worthless as a human being. I was aware that eating junk food and giving in to my cravings made me far worse. If I had some "sinful" foods in the cupboard I would eat them all pre-menstrually, and then tell myself that I deserved to feel awful, because that was all I was fit for. It felt like I was punishing myself. I felt utterly fatigued. I'd go to bed at 8 p.m. each night, feeling dead, and then wake up the next morning feeling equally awful.

I always used to feel I wasn't doing my job properly. I think I inherited this from my mother. Looking back I think she suffered too. There were times when my father would come home to find us throwing things around the kitchen at each other. We'd be fine for a couple of weeks and then it would all start up again.

What about them?

I really hated everybody when I was pre-menstrual. I used to turn my anger on to myself as I couldn't bear to see the effect it had on others. I felt like I literally changed character, like Jekyll and Hyde.

The suicidal feelings I had were both strange and positive. I couldn't talk myself out of them, despite the fact that I really knew, deep down, that suicide was not a good solution. I felt so determined at times, I really felt I would have succeeded if I hadn't been found.

I must emphasize that these feelings and suicidal tendencies only occurred pre-menstrually. I felt utterly dreadful pre-menstrually, like a jibbering wreck.

I think stress aggravated the situation. Both my husband and I are in high-pressure jobs. I've been attending relaxation classes which I find helpful. I don't find it easy to unwind; there is a part of me that remains burning away, probably because I tend to lack confidence and so I'm always pushing myself. I used to burn out at PMS times, but I don't any more.

Apart from all the drugs and sleeping tablets I was given, I also tried diuretics, which were prescribed by my doctor as I used to put on seven pounds (3 kg) pre-menstrually. They helped a little bit initially, but by the end of the day my symptoms would be back and I felt as if I was getting nowhere.

My doctor then prescribed Primolut N in massive doses and all it succeeded in doing was make me gain even more weight. There was a time, five or six years ago, when I tried another hormone treatment, but I didn't get on very well with that either. I felt I was given too much, and it seemed to exaggerate my symptoms. I had a Well Woman test at the time and they said how enlarged my uterus was, and that it was probably due to the hormones.

It was through the media that I learned about the nutritional approach to PMS.'

Anita was a classic case of pure PMS. She had practically no symptoms after her period, and very severe symptoms in all four sub-categories of PMS pre-menstrually, which you can see on her first chart.

Again, from the sound of her symptoms she might well have been classified as a psychiatric patient. After all, screaming in the street in the middle of the night and suicidal feelings are not classified as socially acceptable behaviour.

Although she was taking prescribed sleeping tablets and hormones, she was unable to function properly. Consequently she found it unbelievably difficult to keep herself together at work. It was a wonder she managed to hold down her job at all under the circumstances. You can see how severe these symptoms were from her first chart overleaf.

PRE-MENSTRUAL SYNDROME QUESTIONNAIRE

Name: Anita Walker   Age: 36   Height: 5' 4½"   Weight: 11st

MARITAL STATUS: Single _____ Married _✓_ Divorced _____ Widowed _____
(Please tick where applicable)

PRESENT CONTRACEPTION: None_____ Pill_____ I.U.D. _✓_ Other_____

Your periods come every ___28___ days   Your periods last ___7___ days

Your periods are: Light_____ Moderate_____ Heavy _✓_

Number of Pregnancies: ___4___   Number of Miscarriages: ___2___

Birth weight of children:
1st child _7lb 3oz_ 2nd child _8lb 2oz_ 3rd child_____ 4th child_____

SYMPTOMS	WEEK AFTER PERIOD (Fill in 3 days after period)				WEEK BEFORE PERIOD (Fill in 2-3 days before period)			
	None	Mild	Moderate	Severe	None	Mild	Moderate	Severe
PMS - A								
Nervous Tension	✓							✓
Mood Swings	✓							✓
Irritability	✓							✓
Anxiety	✓							✓
PMS - H								
Weight Gain	✓							✓
Swelling of Extremities			✓					✓
Breast Tenderness	✓							✓
Abdominal Bloating		✓						✓
PMS - C								
Headache	✓						✓	
Craving for Sweets	✓							✓
Increased Appetite	✓							✓
Heart Pounding	✓				✓			
Fatigue	✓							✓
Dizziness or Fainting	✓				✓			
PMS - D								
Depression	✓							✓
Forgetfulness	✓							✓
Crying	✓						✓	
Confusion	✓							✓
Insomnia	✓							✓
OTHER SYMPTOMS								
Loss of Sexual Interest	✓				✓			
Disorientation	✓							✓
Clumsiness	✓							✓
Tremors/Shakes	✓							✓
Thoughts of Suicide	✓							✓
Agoraphobia	✓					✓		
Increased Physical Activity	✓				✓			
Heavy/Aching Legs	✓							✓
Generalized Aches	✓							✓
Bad Breath	✓							✓
Sensitivity to Music/Light	✓				✓			
Excessive Thirst	✓							✓

FOLLOW UP
PRE-MENSTRUAL SYNDROME QUESTIONNAIRE

Name: Anita Walker   Age: 36   Height: 5' 4½"   Weight: 10st 12lb

MARITAL STATUS: Single _____   Married ✓   Divorced _____   Widowed _____
(Please tick where applicable)

PRESENT CONTRACEPTION: None_____   Pill_____   I.U.D. ✓   Other_____

Your periods come every __21__ days   Your periods last __7__ days

Your periods are: Light_____   Moderate ✓   Heavy_____

SYMPTOMS

	WEEK AFTER PERIOD (Fill in 3 days after period)				WEEK BEFORE PERIOD (Fill in 2-3 days before period)			
	None	Mild	Moderate	Severe	None	Mild	Moderate	Severe
PMS - A								
Nervous Tension	✓				✓			
Mood Swings	✓					✓		
Irritability	✓					✓		
Anxiety	✓					✓		
PMS - H								
Weight Gain	✓				✓			
Swelling of Extremities	✓				✓			
Breast Tenderness	✓				✓			
Abdominal Bloating	✓				✓			
PMS - C								
Headache	✓					✓		
Craving for Sweets	✓					✓		
Increased Appetite	✓					✓		
Heart Pounding	✓				✓			
Fatigue	✓					✓		
Dizziness or Fainting	✓				✓			
PMS - D								
Depression	✓				✓			
Forgetfulness	✓				✓			
Crying	✓				✓			
Confusion	✓				✓			
Insomnia	✓					✓		
OTHER SYMPTOMS								
Loss of Sexual Interest	✓					✓		
Disorientation	✓				✓			
Clumsiness	✓					✓		
Tremors/Shakes	✓				✓			
Thoughts of Suicide	✓				✓			
Agoraphobia	✓				✓			
Increased Physical Activity	✓				✓			
Heavy/Aching Legs	✓				✓			
Generalized Aches	✓				✓			
Bad Breath	✓				✓			
Sensitivity to Music/Light	✓				✓			
Excessive Thirst	✓				✓			

'When I began the nutritional PMS programme, I was taking both Primolut N and Mogadon. Very soon after I was able to stop taking both of the drugs. I no longer felt I needed them.

The new diet

I made all the dietary changes suggested and stuck to them rigidly. In fact, I changed the whole family's diet. My son turned out to have some allergies which had been causing behavioural problems. My husband also turned out to have a problem. One day when he was under a lot of stress, he went out to lunch. He ate a lot of bread and pasta and had some alcohol with the meal. On the train on the way home his bladder stopped working and an ambulance had to be called as he was in a terrible state of near-collapse. He was rushed to hospital and was subsequently diagnosed as having a massive dose of thrush. He said it was the most awful thing in his life, the swelling and the irritation were so bad.

I took him off wheat and yeast-based foods and I am now very particular about our diet.

The whole family now look and feel better. You can see it, they sort of "glow" somehow. They are not black around the eyes as they used to be, their hair shines and they have a lot more energy. Maybe that's partly because they have a lot more green vegetables and other fresh raw foods.

We now watch each other's plates and occasionally, if he's suspicious, Mark, my son, will check through my bag!

Come home Mum, all is forgiven

We can actually hold a conversation now. We have good discussions and I really think my family are coming around to thinking I'm a worthwhile person again, probably because I myself consider I am. I can actually say we are back to having a normal married life. David is delighted we live life normally and feels it's great that we are still together, which is lovely. We all joke about my former behaviour. They are much more responsive now, but then again I suppose I am, too.'

After six months Anita had her PMS well and truly under control. She had some remaining mild symptoms which she finds comparatively easy to live with – although within another few months these too should disappear.

The comparison between her two questionnaires clearly shows the progress that Anita felt she made during the six months on the programme, and her letter outlines how her life has since changed.

Dear Maryon,

A very big thank-you to your team for saving a life and a marriage.

As you know, when I wrote to you, I had tried everything I knew and everything my doctor knew to relieve the pain of my PMS. So I wrote to you and will always be glad I did, as the nutritional programme helped so much.

I felt that the hysterectomy without the nutritional programme would not have made such a difference. I can be certain that my speedy recovery was certainly thanks to good nutrition and definitely to the vitamin supplement, Optivite; I took six a day then.

When I wrote to you my only fear was 'What if this fails too?' I almost didn't post the letter when I contemplated the consequences of this: certain divorce, Ben taking the children away because of my emotional instability (and I would have agreed with him) and my certain self-destruction. Happily we can be sure now that this will not happen. As I said, you saved a life and marriage.

Whoever said 'you are what you eat' was so right. I do tend to think I am cured and slip back occasionally to bad eating habits. I then feel tired, cross and lethargic. I suffer this for a day or two and say, look, you're 'going off' again, you're not cured at all. Then I realize what's happening, check back on what I've eaten, and within 36 hours can be all right again; the power of food!

I do enjoy the 'high' of constant energy and health and most of all the joy of not having to take drugs. I will recommend your Service to all who have difficulties. I am battling with my GP at present to recommend his patients to you but he sees it all as 'black magic'. He says I'm better because I think I'm better! He's only got to read my notes. The only time I have seen him since my hysterectomy last year was to talk to him about you. I have not consulted him for anything else.

Again, my thanks and that of my family.

Anita Walker

PAULINE'S SUICIDAL FEELINGS

'One day I felt so awful. I had pre-menstrual insomnia and was desperate to get some sleep. I decided I was going to have a good long sleep. I took all the tablets and then after a while I became panic-stricken and chickened out. I called my husband and told him what I'd done. I can't remember much, except he was trying to keep me awake. When the doctor arrived he said, "We've had problems with you threatening to do this before, haven't we? It's your periods isn't it, you always get like that." This was because I'd said I felt like doing it many times in the past.'

9

OTHER SYMPTOMS –
CLUMSINESS,
LOSS OF SEX DRIVE
AND AGORAPHOBIA

After the first year of providing nutritional help to women, it became obvious that there were other pre-menstrual symptoms that were affecting them severely. We made additions to the chart to assess the most common extra symptoms (see chart overleaf).

CLUMSINESS

Clumsiness was the most troublesome additional symptom to our 1000 patients outside the four sub-groups. Eighty-three per cent of sufferers reported being clumsy pre-menstrually, nearly 56 per cent severe to moderately.

The cause of pre-menstrual clumsiness is uncertain, but it may reflect a disturbance in the finer aspects of nervous system function, which might occur pre-menstrually. This can be caused by changes in brain chemistry, hormonal chemistry, lack of certain nutrients, excessive intake of tea, coffee, cigarettes or alcohol. The presence of pre-menstrual clumsiness suggests that there may well be a substantial physical, rather than psychological, component to such women's pre-menstrual symptoms.

**Degree to which
clumsiness affected
a sample of 1000 women
pre-menstrually**

═══════════════════════

None	Mild	Moderate	Severe	Total Affected
16.6%	27.5%	36.1%	19.8% -	83.4%

SEX DRIVE

Out of a sample of 1000 PMS sufferers with sexual relationships 67 per cent reported decreased interest in sex and frequency of sexual intercourse pre-menstrually. Only 1.5 per cent reported increased sexual activity pre-menstrually.

OTHER SYMPTOMS	WEEK BEFORE PERIOD				WEEK AFTER PERIOD			
Loss of Sexual Interest	✓				✓			
Disorientation	✓				✓			
Clumsiness	✓				✓			
Tremors/Shakes	✓				✓			
Thoughts of Suicide	✓				✓			
Agoraphobia	✓				✓			
Increased Physical Activity	✓				✓			
Heavy/Aching Legs	✓				✓			
Generalized Aches	✓				✓			
Bad Breath	✓				✓			
Sensitivity to Music/Light	✓				✓			
Excessive Thirst	✓				✓			

Do you have any other PRE-MENSTRUAL SYMPTOMS not listed above?

1. _____

2. _____

3. _____

4. _____

5. How much weight do you gain before your period? _____

We were concerned to see such a large number of women reporting similar distressing problems, so we decided to follow the progress of a group of 50 severe PMS sufferers, who also had severely decreased sex drive, through a three-month diet and supplement programme to see whether there was any improvement.

After three months these women were asked whether their interest in sex had altered. Fifty per cent of them reported that there had been a complete return to their libido (sex drive) and a further 38 per cent reported a significant but not full improvement to their libido. Only 12 per cent reported no change in libido at all.

The results were obviously very encouraging. Considering neither we nor the women had anticipated improvement in this area initially, it was considered by all to be an added bonus. In most cases the women did not associate their decreased libido with their PMS, and furthermore did not feel that reduced libido was a symptom, but merely a reflection of the state and stage of their relationship. Needless to say, many husbands and partners were satisfied with this particular result.

Improvement in sex drive of 50 women who had previously reported a decrease

Little or no improvement	Significant but not full return to libido	Complete return of libido		Total improvement
12%	38%	50%	-	88%

" Geraldine's Story "

Geraldine, who explained about her intense chocolate craving problems in the PMS C section, also feels her problems with her relationships and sex life were magnified because of her symptoms.

'My relationship with my husband was definitely affected by my pre-menstrual symptoms. I think, in all fairness, we began going through a sticky patch before I had any of the symptoms, but in those days I didn't lash out and hit him. I'd just get worked up. With PMS I just started hitting out in anger. About the most frustrating thing is that he wouldn't row back. He'd just go quiet and go off, we could never discuss it.

I didn't want him to come anywhere near me pre-menstrually, let alone sexually. I didn't want him to cuddle me, touch me, talk to me or be there. I'd go right into myself and would really rather not have any contact with anyone at all.

A lot of the problems with my husband stem from PMS. I'd feel much worse than crabby, it was unbelievably horrible. The other issues would creep in once I'd started to get worked up, and it became very complex.'

AGORAPHOBIA

On our extended symptom list is the condition of agoraphobia, the exaggerated fear of going out alone. This was eventually added to the list as it seemed to be mentioned far more often than we had anticipated. At about this time we were contacted by a marvellous lady who was running a national group for agoraphobic sufferers. She had some amazing facts and figures about agoraphobia, including statistics on the incidence of PMS-suffering agoraphobic women.

Firstly, we were surprised to learn that 88 per cent of agoraphobia sufferers are women. Out of a sample of 94 agoraphobic women 91 per cent also suffered with PMS!

By coincidence, we had several severe PMS sufferers who also suffered severely with agoraphobia on our programme at this time. Many of them were making excellent progress, not only with the overcoming of their PMS symptoms, but their agoraphobia had also disappeared on the programme.

I'll never forget one joyous phone call I had from a lady in Jersey, who had taken herself out for the day for the first time in eight years. She had gone to have her hair permed and buy some clothes.

As she had previously only gone out accompanied by her husband or a neighbour, when her husband arrived home and found her missing he became understandably worried. After a while he began knocking on neighbours' doors to see whether she had gone visiting. By the time she casually wandered home her husband and neighbours were out in the street looking for her. They couldn't believe her new hair-do, and her husband wasn't sure whether to laugh or cry when he saw how many packages she had! He told me she's been costing him a fortune in evening entertainment ever since! Well, she has got eight years to make up for.

Agoraphobia is a very nasty condition: being afraid to go out is both anti-social and isolating for the victim, and can place an awful strain on a family. Here is the story of a woman who had been perfectly well until she underwent surgery for the purpose of sterilization. The change in her health was so unexpected that it had dramatic repercussions on her life.

" Jane's Story "

Jane was a 36-year-old mother of three children who was trying to work part time at the time she contacted the Women's Nutritional Advisory Service. I say 'trying to work' as for six years she had been severely agoraphobic pre-menstrually.

'It was six years ago that I went to my front door and discovered I couldn't walk through it. I was pre-menstrual at the time, and had noticed symptoms had begun after my sterilization.

I couldn't go out alone, not to the shops or to the bingo, which I had always taken in my stride. I really thought I was suffering from a very serious illness. I saw my doctor and he diagnosed nervous tension. I didn't believe him though, because I'm not the nervous type.

My doctor prescribed Valium, but it was no help. In fact it made me feel worse because it gave me panic attacks. I was on Valium for six months and then had great difficulty stopping. I went back to the doctor when I was pre-menstrual and just threw the tablets at him. I told him to never, ever prescribe me any kind of tablets like that again, as they made me feel so ill.

Previously, I would have been described by my family and friends as practical, hard-working and always full of fun and laughter. I was frightened and bewildered by the changes in myself. I found myself losing new friends as they grew tired of hearing my constant tales of woe.

I was at the doctor's every other week with my list of symptoms. He referred me to a psychiatrist at one point who insisted I was as strong as a horse and that the condition was all in my mind. I was gaining four to five pounds (2–3 kg) in weight pre-menstrually, suffering with severe breast soreness, pounding headaches, edginess and irritability and then the agoraphobia would start. I was sure it wasn't all in my mind.

After recovering from the effects of the Valium I had been taking, we decided to move so that I could be near my supportive family. My new doctor suggested hormone therapy as he said it was usually prescribed for women who were going through the menopause early, but I was only 36 years old! When I read contra-indications of the hormones I decided that as an overweight, over-35 smoker I should not be on these hormones.

I had now reached an impasse. My doctor had given his advice and I had refused to take it. Coincidentally, a few days later I saw an article in the newspaper about Maryon Stewart and the work she was doing at the Women's Nutritional Advisory Service. When I read the article I couldn't believe it. Here was someone describing me and my symptoms, saying that she had helped other people in similar situations.

I was like an old woman at 36

I was suffering three out of every four weeks. I felt very uptight and niggly all the time. Plus I felt really frustrated and frightened that I couldn't get to the bottom of the problem.

The only way I could get out during the day was on the arm of an elderly neighbour in her seventies, who walks with the aid of a walking stick. There was I, half her age, clinging to her. Talk about the blind leading the blind! We'd even have to stop off on the way at my friend's shop because I was shaking so much.

I tried to forget it, but life was far from normal. I began to wonder if I would ever feel right again.

My miserable family

I was sheer hell to live with. For five years I had lived a life of misery and so had my family. My husband was very good, considering what I put him through. I used to deliberately row with him pre-menstrually and pick holes in things. I was very agitated and always looking for an argument. He would avoid me at this time of my cycle. Sexual relations were a real problem in view of how I felt pre-menstrually, plus the fact that I was so tired, I just wasn't up to it.

My husband had to take me everywhere. I was utterly dependent on him. You can't have a normal relationship under these circumstances. But at least I am lucky that he was so supportive.'

Jane's problem areas were PMS A, H and C as well as her agoraphobia. She was literally a shadow of her former self. Her 'before' and 'after' charts and a letter to us are here for you to examine. She also comments on the dietary changes she had to make on the nutritional programme.

Dear Maryon,

As you know, when I first contacted you, I described all my symptoms of PMS. One was of being unable at certain times of the month (i.e. just before and after each period) to leave the house. I experienced severe anxiety and panic attacks going shopping, and doing my evening job was sheer terror with the feeling of passing out, sickness and sweating. Fortunately, my husband took me to and picked me up from the school where I do two hours' cleaning. During the day when I had to go shopping, the feelings were so severe I used to wait for my children to come home from school, then send them to do any shopping I needed.

However, after following your diet recommendations, the attacks lessened to such a degree I go out now without even thinking about it.

I started a new part-time office job. It started a day before my period was due and yet that week I didn't experience any problems at all. I went to town shopping after work, came home, cooked, cleaned, did my evening job and although I felt tired, at no time did I suffer from any feelings of panic or anxiety.

I went completely off the diet and ate and drank all the things I shouldn't have: within 48 hours I suffered really bad stomach ache and diarrhoea. All the feelings returned, so I am now back sticking strictly to

PRE-MENSTRUAL SYNDROME QUESTIONNAIRE

Name: Jane Moor   Age: 36   Height: 5' 6"   Weight: 11st 11lb

MARITAL STATUS: Single _____   Married _✓_   Divorced _____   Widowed _____
(Please tick where applicable)

PRESENT CONTRACEPTION: None _✓_   Pill_____   I.U.D. _____   Other _____

 Your periods come every 26–30 days   Your periods last   4   days

 Your periods are: Light __✓__   Moderate_____   Heavy_____

 Number of Pregnancies: 3   Number of Miscarriages: __–__

Birth weight of children:
 1st child_____   2nd child •_____   3rd child_____   4th child_____

SYMPTOMS	WEEK AFTER PERIOD (Fill in 3 days after period)				WEEK BEFORE PERIOD (Fill in 2-3 days before period)			
	None	Mild	Moderate	Severe	None	Mild	Moderate	Severe
PMS - A								
Nervous Tension	✓						✓	
Mood Swings	✓						✓	
Irritability		✓						✓
Anxiety			✓					✓
PMS - H								
Weight Gain	✓						✓	
Swelling of Extremities	✓					✓		
Breast Tenderness	✓							✓
Abdominal Bloating	✓							✓
PMS - C								
Headache			✓					✓
Craving for Sweets	✓					✓		
Increased Appetite	✓					✓		
Heart Pounding	✓						✓	
Fatigue	✓							✓
Dizziness or Fainting			✓				✓	
PMS - D								
Depression	✓					✓		
Forgetfulness	✓				✓			
Crying	✓				✓			
Confusion	✓				✓			
Insomnia	✓						✓	
OTHER SYMPTOMS								
Loss of Sexual Interest			✓				✓	
Disorientation	✓				✓			
Clumsiness			✓				✓	
Tremors/Shakes		✓				✓		
Thoughts of Suicide	✓				✓			
Agoraphobia			✓					✓
Increased Physical Activity	✓					✓		
Heavy/Aching Legs	✓						✓	
Generalized Aches	✓						✓	
Bad Breath	✓				✓			
Sensitivity to Music/Light	✓				✓			
Excessive Thirst	✓				✓			

FOLLOW UP
PRE-MENSTRUAL SYNDROME QUESTIONNAIRE

Name: Jane Moor   Age: 36   Height: 5' 6"   Weight: 11st 5lb

MARITAL STATUS: Single _____ Married _√_ Divorced _____ Widowed _____
(Please tick where applicable)

PRESENT CONTRACEPTION: None _√_ Pill_____ I.U.D. _____ Other_____

   Your periods come every _26–30_ days   Your periods last _4_ days

   Your periods are: Light _√_ Moderate_____ Heavy_____

SYMPTOMS

	WEEK AFTER PERIOD (Fill in 3 days after period)				WEEK BEFORE PERIOD (Fill in 2-3 days before period)			
	None	Mild	Moderate	Severe	None	Mild	Moderate	Severe
PMS - A								
Nervous Tension	√				√			
Mood Swings	√				√			
Irritability	√					√		
Anxiety	√				√			
PMS - H								
Weight Gain	√					√		
Swelling of Extremities	√				√			
Breast Tenderness	√					√		
Abdominal Bloating	√					√		
PMS - C								
Headache	√				√			
Craving for Sweets	√					√		
Increased Appetite	√				√			
Heart Pounding	√				√			
Fatigue	√					√		
Dizziness or Fainting	√				√			
PMS - D								
Depression	√				√			
Forgetfulness	√				√			
Crying	√				√			
Confusion	√				√			
Insomnia	√				√			
OTHER SYMPTOMS								
Loss of Sexual Interest	√				√			
Disorientation	√				√			
Clumsiness	√				√			
Tremors/Shakes	√				√			
Thoughts of Suicide	√				√			
Agoraphobia	√					√		
Increased Physical Activity	√					√		
Heavy/Aching Legs	√					√		
Generalized Aches	√					√		
Bad Breath	√				√			
Sensitivity to Music/Light	√				√			
Excessive Thirst	√				√			

your diet. Although I still have a queasy tum and headache, I can see myself getting back to normal.

The diet really works, I feel a new woman after six years of living in sheer hell.

Jane Moor

Dietary changes

'I already knew I was allergic to eggs when I began the programme. It seems to run in my family. I was astonished, though, to be asked to give up all grains execpt brown rice, all sugar, tea and coffee and reduce my intake of dairy products.

I followed the diet rigidly for the first three months I felt on top of the world. I lost weight, which was great, and was able to go out alone for the first time in six years. I got so much better that I am now able to hold down a full-time job. I have let the diet slip a bit more recently. You tend to take it all for granted when you are feeling really well. Plus it takes extra time and effort shopping for and preparing special food. I know that once I tighten my diet up again I will feel 100 per cent again.'

All Jane's long-standing severe symptoms either cleared up completely or became very mild and 'livable' with. Diet was a major factor in her case, as she has proved to herself.

CRIME OR ILLNESS?

Finally in this section, I return to the subject of violence. As violence in general is on the increase in our society I feel this is an area which is certainly worthy of fuller discussion.

As early as 1845 menstrually-related disorders were accepted by the courts as a defence for a criminal act. In that year there were three recorded examples:

- Martha, a servant who, without motive, murdered her employer's child, was acquitted on the grounds of insanity caused by 'obstructed menstruation'.

- A woman was acquitted of murdering her young niece on the grounds of insanity stemming from disordered menstruation.

- A woman servant was accused of theft and was acquitted at Carlisle quarter sessions on the grounds of temporary insanity 'from suppression of the menses'.

So you see, it's not such a new problem. We probably talk openly about it now, whereas years ago it would have been hushed up. More recently there have been other famous cases where PMS has been a large part of the defence.

Dr Dalton reported in *The Lancet* in 1980 the case of a 28-year-old worker in the food industry who was accused of fatally stabbing her girlfriend. Following the stabbing she was admitted to prison and noted to be menstruating. Although she was imprisoned, it was acknowledged that she had severe PMS which was subsequently treated. In 1982 she was freed on probation on the grounds of PMS.

There have been several other similar cases over the past few years. There was the case of Anna Reynolds who battered her mother to death in June 1986. She was convicted of murder in February 1987, and subsequently at appeal the charge was reduced to manslaughter on the basis of diminished responsibility whilst suffering with Pre-Menstrual Syndrome. Debra Lovell was another victim of PMS who became a human fireball after soaking herself in paraffin whilst she was pre-menstrual.

In November 1988 a teenage mother, Donna Kelly, suffering from PMS unintentionally killed her seven-week-old son by shaking him when he would not stop crying. The verdict recorded was not guilty as it was appreciated that Donna Kelly had previously been a loving mother who did not have the intention to kill her baby.

In May 1989 a mother of four killed her son after he 'wound her up'. She walked free from the Old Bailey after the judge said she was sick, rather than evil.

And then there was the case of Nicola Owen who made medical and legal history by becoming the first woman successfully to use PMS as a mitigating plea in the courts, when she was discharged from the Old Bailey where she faced arson charges.

This evidence that some women become more vulnerable, unpredictable and even lose control pre-menstrually and around the time of the onset of their period, confirms the fact that the Pre-Menstrual Syndrome is a common condition which can be life-threatening and should most certainly be taken seriously.

It does, however, mean that PMS may be considered a plausible excuse for an offence. This, I am only too aware, is a very sensitive subject. Like any other scapegoat, it has and will, I'm sure, continue to be used in the courts as a means of reducing or escaping sentence.

Although, at the Women's Nutritional Advisory Service, we have encountered our share of criminal cases, I feel it is important to take a stand on this issue. There is no way that we condone any crime, or believe that a woman should be excused for her actions due to PMS. However, it is acknowledged that PMS can be a contributing factor which should be considered along with all the other factors in each individual case.

Each person, be they male or female, has the responsibility to look after their own body. There is evidence now, for example, that indicates that poor diet is related to delinquency and even dyslexia.

Rather than excusing women with PMS for their actions, or adolescents who offend for their behaviour, it would be better to help them overcome the problem by at least correcting their nutritional state. The upsetting and frustrating fact is that much education is needed, both for the public and also for the medical profession. Just knowing which foods help and which foods may harm would be a great start. Having some basic understanding of how diet can affect one's state of mind, for instance, would be invaluable.

We hope that over the next few years doctors will be taking all this into consideration, much more so than they are generally doing at present.

In the meantime, the courts have the difficult task of deciding where to draw the line. There should certainly be the facility for them to check on a woman's nutritional state and have her assessed for PMS. This assessment usually would take three months to confirm as three consecutive cycles need to be charted in order to confirm the diagnosis of PMS.

The fact that a woman may be a danger to herself or society has to be dealt with in a routine way by the courts. When PMS is presented as a defence or mitigation, and the diagnosis confirmed, then effective treatment should be sought whilst the woman is serving her sentence, if she has been convicted.

It is very important that when PMS is used as a defence or mitigation, appropriate treatment is instituted. It then becomes the woman's personal responsibility to follow the appropriate diet or take the appropriate treatment to ensure that her pre-menstrual symptoms are properly controlled. PMS could then not be used as a defence or mitigation should she then re-offend.

10

THE SOCIAL
IMPLICATIONS
OF PMS

RELATIONSHIPS AT HOME AND AT WORK

It was not surprising that as a result of these severe symptoms, we were recording that 95 per cent of our survey of women reported that their home lives and relationships with family and friends were affected by their PMS symptoms.

Degree to which a sample of 1000 women felt that their home life/relationship with family/friends was affected due to PMS symptoms

Not Affected	Mild	Moderate	Severe	Total Affected
4.9%	12.7%	36.1%	46.3% -	95.1%

You will have read in earlier sections about how some family lives were affected. I have added two quite different examples here to make the point

in its own right, as the family and our immediate circle are so very important.

Anita, who suffered severely with all four sub-groups, and actually
attempted suicide, explains how she felt her home life was affected.

ANITA'S PROBLEMS AT HOME

'From about 1982 I used to get so bad-tempered. I remember one day I
was having an ordinary discussion with my husband and he made a
comment which I took the wrong way. I started attacking him with a
knife. Then I'd start attacking everybody else in the house except the
baby, who I made a point of keeping away from.

I firmly believe that if we hadn't been having difficulties with our son at
the time, my husband would have left me. I think he had got to the point
where he couldn't take any more. My marriage was really under severe
pressure. He was definitely on the point of saying "That's it".

I have two children and I think they have both been affected by my pre-
menstrual behaviour. They learned to watch me carefully to see the mood
I was in. This is because I would often attack them verbally and be cruel.
Then afterwards I would pick them up and cuddle them. I couldn't always
keep myself under control. They didn't understand. I think they have
forgiven me now, but they still watch me. I don't think they can believe
I'm not going to flip on them.'

Geraldine, whose worst problem was her secret chocolate binges, took her
anger and frustration out on her daughters.

GERALDINE'S FEELINGS OF ANGER

'I feel really aggressive towards the children, especially the older ones. I
smack them in instances where it's not really deserved. I tend to take it
out on the oldest daughter, even if she hasn't done anything to justify it.

The worst thing with the children is not so much the aggressiveness,
because when I feel that way I try to keep away from them, but the
sarcasm. I can be really horrible, and it's awful because it takes away all
their self-confidence.

After being really awful I'd just go into the bedroom and lean my head
on the wall and think, "Fancy saying something like that?" I'd feel really

wicked and go into floods of tears. Sometimes I'd blame them and ask them how they could do this to me. I'd tell them that they were making me ill and accuse them of being horrid to me. Then I'd complain that they didn't do a thing around the house and threaten to get a maid. By this time they would be staring at me, absolutely rigid with fright. All the time, at the back of my mind I'd know I was being a bitch and feel crumby, really crumby because basically I love my girls to death and I don't want to say such awful things to them.'

PERSONAL RELATIONSHIPS

It is exceedingly difficult to maintain a loving relationship when you are experiencing severe symptoms of irritability, nervous tension and aggression. I so often see women whose personal and sexual relationships have fallen apart as a direct result of their PMS. Penny and Liz are two good examples of how symptoms stood in the way of a harmonious personal life. The good news is that they both, like the majority of our patients, were able to restore their relationships once over their symptoms. It is not uncommon for men to thank us for giving them back the girl they married!

" Penny's Story "

Penny is a 40-year-old director of a small publishing and public relations company who works and lives with her partner.

'I knew that unless I took some drastic action, I would lose my boyfriend. My ex-husband used to take the stance of ignoring me until the mood was over. However, John would not accept that I would be so moody with him one minute and then pick up the telephone and speak perfectly normally to clients. At work I seemed to be able to control myself for short periods of time. I was able to switch on this false smile and air of calmness. But once amongst those I loved and trusted, I'd let rip about how I really felt inside. When John first moved in with me he was staggered to discover the effect that PMS had on me. At first he tried to arrange business trips away to coincide with my PMS days, but because my cycle was irregular planning them wasn't easy.

Our relationship nearly snapped

Each month it was as if the normal, happy me disappeared for up to ten days, and was replaced by an irritable, moody and very clumsy woman. My PMS symptoms nearly broke up our relationship. I'd snap at John and be really rude when his children came to visit.

I knew from early on that I was suffering from PMS. It started when I stopped taking the contraceptive pill when I was 33. In desperation I tried all the remedies I'd read about, but they made no difference at all. Then I spotted an article suggesting that PMS could be helped by diet. I was very sceptical, but concerned enough about my relationship with John to give it a try.

Diet brought me back to normal

I followed the diet that was tailor-made for me, took specific vitamin and mineral supplements, and did some moderate exercise. It took three months to overcome my symptoms. The moodiness and snappiness subsided, and thankfully I was normal and happy all the time again.

John and I are now on an even keel.'

John is obviously delighted that Penny found a solution, and feels that PMS affects men every bit as much as it does women. He says, 'Having been through some tough times at the start, I'm convinced that many marriages must fail not because the couple aren't right together, but because PMS comes between them.'

❝ Liz's Story ❞

'I suffered with PMS for about four years and was gradually worsening. It became so bad I sought help from my GP. The worst symptoms I suffered were mainly terrible food cravings - particularly for sweet things. I could go through not just one bar of chocolate but half a dozen at one sitting. That made me feel terribly bloated abdominally, I had terrible breast tenderness and I felt really really depressed.

I don't know how he put up with me!

My PMS symptoms affected the relationship I have with my husband on a month to month basis – in between times I would be fine, but at that time of the month I would completely change and because of my mood swings and depression it did put a strain on things. I didn't want to cook, I didn't want to go out – I was really withdrawn into myself. I could go from being happy one minute and dress to go out, and because I was so bloated and my skirt wouldn't fasten, I would stomp into a rage and I just wasn't going out and it wasn't for discussion. I don't know how he put up with me – he was very supportive, but it did put a great strain on things.

I tried various treatments from vitamin B6 tablets to water tablets and I eventually went on to hormone therapy, none of which I found very helpful at all. I really didn't want to be taking drug treatment in the long term. I was more interested in finding a more natural method but did not seem to find it through my GP.

When I followed the Women's Nutritional Advisory Service programme that was sent to me through the post, and I followed all the recommendations I received over the telephone, there was a vast difference even within the first month. I followed the programme for about six months and got continued help and support from the telephone helpline and by letter. Any problems I had, or any worrying symptoms, I could just phone up and chat things through.

I'm feeling a lot better now. I'm virtually symptom-free. I carried on with the diet, the exercise and the supplements, and I'm really, really grateful for the help and support I was given by the WNAS.'

PRODUCTIVITY AND EFFICIENCY AT WORK

Another incredible statistic that emerged from the study on 1000 PMS sufferers was the degree to which their work suffered as a result of their symptoms. 92.7 per cent reported that their productivity and efficiency decreased pre-menstrually.

They further reported that they were, to a large degree, 'not there mentally' for an average of five days per month! This means that they produce very little work during this period of time.

" Ifey's Story "

Ifey is a 29-year-old barrister who suffered with PMS for 17 years.

'My worst PMS symptoms were nausea. I always felt nausea and in the latter years I would be continuously vomiting, which I found the hardest thing to deal with. Apart from that I used to feel very depressed. I'd be very weepy, upset and emotional for no apparent reason. I used to put on weight and become very bloated.

PMS affected my work

I always felt I wasn't functioning properly and wasn't doing my best workwise. I'm a barrister and I need to be able to concentrate and I need to be able to think very quickly, but when I was suffering from my symptoms, I wasn't able to do that and consequently it affected my work. I'd always hope that when my symptoms came I had a case that was easy to deal with and didn't involve a lot of work or concentration.

Altogether I had suffered with PMS for 17 years. I had been to several gynaecologists to get help with my symptoms. Initially my GP had told me that I would continue to have these symptoms until I had my first child; since I started my period when I was 11 that wasn't very helpful. I was put on the pill at the age of 16 and I took the pill for 10 years to deal with the symptoms; but it wasn't very helpful. It was only helpful in so much as it would suppress symptoms during exam times.

My symptoms vanished overnight

When I went on the PMS programme I was told I would have to cut out chocolate from my diet, which I found very hard because I love chocolate. Also I was told to avoid foods containing wheat and alcohol before my symptoms arrived, to exercise and to take the recommended supplements. Having done that for a month, and I stuck regularly to the programme, my symptoms just vanished overnight. It was just absolutely amazing. Normally the symptoms would be there, but I had no symptoms whatsoever, it was just like a miracle, and after 17 years of suffering it was just brilliant!'

A labour force survey conducted in 1992 found that there were just over 11 million working women in the UK. Over nine million were employed and the remainder were self-employed. Given these figures the cost to industry due to lack of production must be vast, and probably not a statistic that has been properly considered. It wouldn't register as sickness or absenteeism as these women appear to be at work in the normal way. Unless specifically asked for, this information would not appear. Indeed, even asking for it may not produce the truth as there are so many women who would be in fear of losing their jobs. As it is, they feel they are teetering on the edge of disaster at work because of their general behaviour pre-menstrually. **81.6 per cent** of 1000 women felt that their work or career had been adversely affected by their PMS. So keeping a low profile is the least line of resistance.

Effects on productivity/efficiency pre-menstrually out of a sample of 1000 women		
Same	*Decreased*	*Increased*
6.2%	92.7%	1.1%

In 1993 the results of a study we undertook on work efficiency were published. It was to my knowledge the first study of its kind in the UK. In conjunction with Kimberly-Clark, the makers of Kleenex and Simplicity products, we were able to work with 47 of their staff who were suffering with PMS. The group was split into two, with half the women making dietary changes and taking Optivite, and the other half just making dietary changes. There was an improvement in work efficiency in both groups with a trend towards increased benefit in the group taking the nutritional supplement as well. As a group all the women reported an increased sense of well-being and energy levels.

A look at case histories of women who came to the Women's Nutritional Advisory Service proves the point. First there was Sally, a divorcee in an executive position.

" Sally's Story "

'I have a very responsible, full-time position. My job involves dealing with people and quite a lot of travel. I found it very difficult to cope pre-menstrually. I felt emotionally unstable and frightened to go out of the house. It made me a liability, really. The moods I experienced gave me feelings of dislike for people I worked with for no apparent reason. Especially my manager.

I would be extremely bad-tempered and unable to concentrate. I had this persecution complex and felt that everybody was against me and scheming. If something went wrong I felt that it was other people's fault and that they were getting at me.

I would sometimes think "sod the lot of them, it's all their fault". I'd try to work, feeling so agitated and ill. I pushed myself to work even harder and faster, which made me even more tired and exhausted.'

Anita, a PMS D sufferer who had attempted suicide, had more than her share of problems at work.

" Anita's Story "

'My work was certainly affected. I would forget things. Forget appointments and forget to put things in the diary. I just couldn't concentrate for that time of the month. In fact I was only normal for one week in four. For three weeks I'd feel so tired and work would take me much longer than usual. It would take me one to two hours to do half-an-hour's work. Consequently, for at least two weeks per month I'd have to work late to get my work done. Even then I'd still have to check all the work again when I wasn't pre-menstrual.'

DRIVING ABILITY

Many of the symptoms discussed have broad repercussions on the sufferer herself and on her family and friends. However, the seriousness of PMS comes right home when a statistic appears that could affect us all. We asked 1000 drivers who suffer with PMS whether their driving ability was affected pre-menstrually. An astounding **76.9 per cent** said their driving ability decreased before their period. Many women stop driving before their period is due as they have previously had so many accidents pre-menstrually. The two main factors that seem to affect driving ability are lack of concentration and poor coordination. Amazingly, the women report that as soon as their period arrives, their driving ability returns to normal.

Driving a car, or any vehicle for that matter, is a real responsibility and not to be taken lightly. We advise severe sufferers to keep off the road until their symptoms have gone, or are under control. Placing lives at risk is no joke. Here are two examples of many who experienced diminished driving skills pre-menstrually.

" Anita's Story "

'I have had several accidents and near-misses, all of which were during my pre-menstrual time. Once, when I was delivering a parcel, I went straight into the back of the car in front of me which was stationary. I didn't even see that he had stopped. Another time I was going to turn right, I saw something coming in the opposite direction and yet I carried on despite the fact that I'd seen the chap. I knew I hadn't got the speed to get past him, but I carried on nevertheless. I made lots of stupid decisions because I didn't have my mind on what was going on around me. I felt very vague and as if I was driving along in a metal box detached from reality. I have an excess on my insurance policy as a result of these accidents.'

" Ruth's Story "

'If I was feeling aggressive generally pre-menstrually, then I would be aggressive behind the wheel. I can remember once, there was a stupid man in a van in front of me at a junction. He was over the white line on the middle of the road. He was going right and I was going left, I was feeling all steamed up. I was alone in the car. I mounted the pavement to get past him, revving up hard and hooting the horn. In fact I scraped my car all along his mudguard. Then I zoomed off. That was typical of how I used to feel. I have still got the car with the mark.'

11

WHY IS PMS MORE COMMON TODAY?

As I have already mentioned, PMS seems to be more common today than in years past. This is undoubtedly partly because it is talked about now in a way that was inconceivable 30 or 40 years ago. But it is probably also due to changes in our lifestyle, diet and possibly our use of hormones and drugs. It is extremely hard to pinpoint any one factor as being a clear-cut cause of PMS. But though the case may not be proven, it may be useful to look at some of these factors and their relationship with PMS and other common diseases that have become the hallmark of the twentieth century.

It is estimated that in 1993 the NHS bill for the taxpayer was £37 billion. In the USA in the last 20 or so years, the medical bill has increased from $27 billion to over $200 billion! The awful fact is that, despite these amounts of money being spent, some of us have been getting sicker.

Cardiovascular disease is still the biggest killer in developed countries and undoubtedly the commonest preventable cause of early death in young to middle-aged men and women. Approximately 170,000 people die each year in the United Kingdom from heart attacks and strokes. There has been little improvement, as yet, in these figures, though the United States and Finland have begun to achieve a substantial fall in their incidences of heart disease. Smoking, lack of exercise, obesity, high blood pressure and high blood cholesterol are all well-documented risk factors and these last three are all influenced by diet.

Cancer too, it appears, is on the increase. There seem to be three main factors for this. The first is age. With a few exceptions the incidence of most cancers rises steeply with age from about 40 years onward. In times past many people did not live long enough to be at risk of developing cancer. Secondly, it is highly likely that there has been a true increase in the rate of cancer this century, regardless of age, and that this reflects the increased use of chemicals in the environment. Many industrial chemicals, pesticides and even drugs linger in the environment for years. Finally, the type of food we eat also influences cancer risk. Consumption of smoked and pickled foods is associated with an increase in some cancers, especially of the stomach and oesophagus, whilst a high intake of fresh fruit and vegetables may well protect against many types of cancer. These protective foods are rich in vitamin C, E and carotene – vegetable vitamin A – which help limit the damage to tissues by cancer-inducing chemicals.

'Mental' illnesses are also on the increase and this too may be influenced by our diet, consumption of alcohol, medical and illicit drugs. Obviously social factors, education and life skills are also all important in helping us cope with times of stress or ill-health. The stresses and strains of twentieth-century living have not made it easy for some of us to cope, and for many women, working and raising a family is particularly stressful.

Allergic problems have also become much more common in the last 40 years. The reasons for this are not clear but include family or genetic factors, chemicals in the environment, dietary habits and the pattern of feeding in childhood.

What, I hear you ask, has this pessimistic view of the state of our health got to do with PMS? Quite simply, it appears that the development of PMS is very much influenced by the same factors: diet, exercise or lack of it, and possibly environmental chemicals. It is possible that these diverse conditions have common causative and aggravating factors.

In 1986 the Women's Nutritional Advisory Service completed a national street survey on 500 women in Britain. We found that 73.6 per cent of them suffered in varying degrees with PMS. This figure is considerably more than estimates of 30–60 per cent made during the previous 30 years.

By now you must be wondering why the diseases are becoming more common, and you might well ask. Our twentieth-century lifestyle brings many relatively new experiences to us, some of which we are not well equipped to handle. The diets most of us know are very far removed from that of our ancestors. Our bodies were not built to cope with refined and processed foods, very often empty of nutrients. We have had to live with pesticides and insecticides being sprayed on our crops, growth hormones and antibiotics pumped into animals, and environmental pollution and acid rain as the finishing touches. Many of us over-eat and under-exercise, and women nowadays tend to lead far more stressful existences. So it is

logical, really, that we can't honestly expect our 'machines' to go on in-
definitely without breaking down when we don't treat them with respect.
We generally treat our cars better than we do our bodies – you wouldn't
dream of putting the wrong fuel in your petrol tank, would you?

Before I launch into the tale of woe about our diet, let me say that
although you will probably come to realize that we are faced with certain
problems concerning our diet, with good education we *can* find ways
around them. I will of course be discussing various solutions in the Self-
Help section on diet in Part Three.

A GOOD LOOK AT OUR DIET

In order to look at diet more closely we need to examine how our habits
have changed during this century.

- We have increased our consumption of sugar. The UK has become
  one of the world's largest chocolate and sweet eaters, with the average
  person consuming some 188 lb or 85 kilos each per year. We currently
  spend over £4 billion per year on chocolate alone.

- Our diet is particularly high in saturated fats (animal fats). It is
  thought that this has much to do with our also having a high incidence of heart disease and breast cancer.

- We eat far too much salt – 10 to 20 times more than our bodies really
  require per day. Salt can contribute to blood pressure problems and
  pre-menstrual water retention.

- We often drink far too much coffee and tea which can impede the
  absorption of essential nutrients. On average we consume four cups of
  tea and two cups of coffee per day, but many people exceed this.

- We consume volumes of foods with a high level of phosphorus, which
  again impedes absorption of good nutrients. Examples of these foods
  are soft drinks of low or normal calorie types, processed foods, canned,
  packaged, pre-packed, convenience foods and ready-made sauces.

- Alcohol consumption has almost doubled in the United Kingdom
  since the end of the Second World War. On average, women drink
  about the equivalent of one unit per day (equal to one glass of wine).
  Not much, you may think, but enough to have a slight adverse effect

on the outcome of pregnancy! Also, about one-third of women are teetotal or consume very little alcohol so someone is having their share.

- Unbelievable as it may seem, we actually eat less food than we did thirty and more years ago. It seems that women of today actually expend less energy than those of a generation or two ago and this has resulted in a 10 to 15 per cent reduction in food intake. This means that our intake of essential nutrients has also fallen, particularly if we eat refined or convenience foods. The motor car and lack of exercise has almost certainly been a factor in the decline in energy expenditure.

- Many of the foods available contain chemical additives in the form of flavour enhancers, colouring and preservatives. Whilst some of these are not harmful, some of them *are*, and our bodies are certainly not designed to cope with them.

- Our water contains certain pollutants which are thought to be a risk to public health.

- Our meat has become contaminated with antibiotics and growth hormones.

- Nitrate fertilizers have been used to obtain fast-growing and abundant crops. It is now recognized that nitrates are harmful and can produce cancer, at least in animals.

- Almost all of our fresh fruit, cereals and vegetables are sprayed with pesticides at least once. In addition, milk and meat may retain the pesticides from feed given to livestock.

Smoking

Smoking tobacco has become a widespread habit among Western societies. In 1922 in the United Kingdom, for example, 20–34-year-old women smoked an average of fifty cigarettes per year, but by 1975 this had risen to an average of just over three thousand cigarettes per woman, per year. Despite the more educated classes reducing their cigarette consumption, smoking has become relatively more common amongst women, in those who are less well educated.

Alcohol

Since the 1940s alcohol consumption has doubled in the United Kingdom. On average, women consume one unit of alcohol per day, and men three units (one unit = 1 glass of wine, 1 pub measure of spirits, 1 small sherry or vermouth, or half a pint of normal strength beer or lager). These average levels are now the maximum recommended daily intakes for women and men respectively. Whilst many of us may be teetotallers, or drink substantially less than this, there will be those who regularly consume more. Some women may go on pre-menstrual alcohol binges.

For every £1 spent on food in the United Kingdom, some 75p is spent on alcohol and tobacco. Just think how the quality of the food in the United Kingdom could improve if only half the money spent on alcohol and tobacco was spent on purchasing better quality food.

Drugs

Western societies have become drug-oriented. In the 12 months of 1991 in the United States nearly £35 billion was spent on medicines by a population of 250 million, and in the UK it was £3.5 billion or £69 per man woman and child. Doctors issue some 15 per cent more prescriptions than they did a decade ago. In England only, over 425 million prescriptions were written in 1992, nearly 10 million for anti-depressants, amounting to £81 million. Not surprising in view of the power and influence that drug companies have been allowed to assume in the education of doctors.

In the last year there has been tremendous concern by medical practitioners worldwide about the excessive use of benzodiazepene tranquillizers and sleeping tablets. It is now recommended that these drugs, which include Valium, Mogadon and Ativan, are used as a temporary measure for only a few weeks. Those who have been taking them long-term should, if at all possible, have their dosage and frequency gradually reduced under medical supervision.

The Pill

The oral contraceptive birth control pill has been a popular and effective method of contraception. The initial forms of the birth pill had high levels of oestrogen, which were known to cause some disturbance in vitamin and mineral balance, increase the risk of vaginal thrush, and in some women precipitate significant depression and migraine headaches. These side-effects are less likely with the new lower dose, or phased dosage oral contraceptive pill. However, problems can certainly arise. Whilst the oral contraceptive pill can help some women's pre-menstrual symptoms, and is a useful way for treating mild PMS, particularly in those women who require contraception, it can also aggravate some PMS symptoms. There is no way of determining this, other than by trial and error. If you find an oral contraceptive pill that suits you, all well and good. However, some women will find that practically any form of the Pill aggravates their premenstrual symptoms.

Vitamin and mineral intake

Our diet this century has gone through, and continues to go through, several substantial changes. By the end of the 1970s there was evidence, from certain surveys, of a deterioration in the quality of the UK diet, particularly since the Second World War. A high intake of sugar, refined foods, animal fats and alcohol had meant a relatively poor intake of essential vitamins and minerals.

Some fifteen vitamins, twenty-four minerals and eight amino acids have been isolated as being essential for normal body function. They are synergistic, which means that they rely upon each other in order to keep the body functioning at an optimum level. When one or more is in short supply, alterations in body metabolism occur. Minor deficiencies can often be tolerated, but major or multiple deficiencies result in the body becoming inefficient, whith the development of symptoms and possibly disease.

There is, however, some heartening recent evidence. All the good advice from numerous individual experts and expert committees, government ones included, has finally got through to *some* of the British public. Many of us have increased our intake of fruit and vegetables and this greatly offsets the potential fall in intake from eating refined foods or eating smaller amounts of food in general. However, this has not happened with the unemployed or those who come from families where the main wage-earner is unskilled. From the recent dietary survey of British adults in the UK, the single biggest factor that determined nutrient intake was not age, sex, illness, or whether on a diet or not, but whether the person was unemployed. Like it or not, it seems that we already have a nutritional underclass who don't have the money and the knowledge to improve their diets. Fats and sugar are cheap calories, and when you are hungry calories are more important than fibre or vitamins and minerals.

Let us now turn our attention to certain specific nutrients which may contribute to symptoms of PMS.

THE NITTY GRITTY REVIEW
OF SPECIFIC NUTRIENTS

Some nutritional factors may be of particular importance to PMS. In the United Kingdom, the Department of Health has instructed the Committee on the Medical Aspects of Food to investigate the nature of the UK diet, and what the appropriate intakes of calories, fats, fibre, vitamins and minerals should be. A similar governmental review by the Food and Drug Administration in the USA was also undertaken in the 1980s.

In 1991 the Department of Health in the UK published its report on Dietary Reference Values for Food Energy and Nutrients for the United Kingdom. This report was prepared by an august group of scientists and doctors who set guidelines for intakes for most of the known essential nutrients. It followed another important report, The Dietary and Nutritional Survey of British Adults. These two reports and similar reports from the United States have allowed a more detailed assessment than ever before of the nutritional adequacy for the adult population in these two developed countries.

Vitamin B

The B group of vitamins, and in particular vitamin B6, have been used for many years to treat PMS. In the UK the new recommended average intake for women of child-bearing age is 1.2 mg per day, exactly the level found in an independent nutrition survey (the Booker Health Report 1985) and less than the value of 1.7 mg from the recent government survey. According to these figures, hardly anyone should be deficient in this nutrient. But several surveys using blood tests have revealed that some 10 to 20 per cent of adults, especially women, appear to have a mild deficiency. This seems more likely in those with problems such as depression and anxiety, as well as PMS. However, deficiency of this nutrient does not explain PMS as many of those with a mild deficiency have no symptoms at all.

Folic acid, another of the B vitamins, was found to be slightly low in between eight and 40 per cent of adult women. Young women seemed particularly at risk. These figures are almost certainly an overestimate of the problem and comparable surveys from the US give values less than half these, but still with no cause for complacency.

Deficiency of these two B group vitamins and the others (B1, B2, B3 and B12), which occur less frequently, can all affect energy level, mood, skin quality, hormone function and appetite. A poor intake may contribute in part to some women's PMS. Certain aspects of our modern diet deserve further comment.

99

Many refined foods are low in B complex vitamins. For example, a McDonald's Big Mac hamburger is known to contain only a fraction of the vitamin B6 that it should do. Presumably, substantial quantities are lost in preparation, cooking and storage. In fact, you would have to eat sixty Big Mac hamburgers a day, in order to achieve an intake of 1.2 mg of vitamin B6 – a current conservative allowance.

Thus, for some of us whose diets do not contain good quantities of fresh and wholesome foods, the intake of B vitamins may be low.

Magnesium

Magnesium is a key mineral in the treatment of PMS. It has now been shown in several medical studies that women with PMS have low levels of magnesium in their red blood cells, and finding a mildly reduced level of magnesium in the blood is now the most consistent reported abnormal finding in women with PMS. Once again, however, not all women with a low level of blood magnesium will have PMS.

Intakes of this mineral in the UK are generally below optimum levels: aproximately 15 per cent of all women in the UK of child-bearing age eat a diet deficient in magnesium, and many others consume only borderline amounts – a low intake (i.e. likely to lead to deficiency) has been defined in the UK as less than 150 mg per day; the recommended intakes and actual intakes in the United States are higher but without any cause for complacency. It may come as no surprise to you to learn that vegetables, fruit and all unrefined or unprocessed foods are rich in this mineral and that refined foods are poor sources. Eating a diet low in protein and high in salt, sugar, alcohol and possibly coffee may contribute to increased losses of magnesium. Like the B vitamins, magnesium has an effect on energy production, mood, muscle function and hormone metabolism. Curiously there are no physical or skin signs of a deficiency.

Magnesium is definitely an important piece of the puzzle of PMS.

Iron

It is probably better known that menstruating women have an increased need for the mineral iron; in fact, iron levels are at their lowest four days pre-menstrually. This time there *is* an RDA (Recommended Daily Allowance) in the UK for iron, which is 12 mg per day; this is somewhat lower than the RDA for the USA, which is 18 mg.

The Booker Health Report showed that 60 per cent of females between the ages of 18 and 54 have iron levels below the recommended daily allowance. In another study in 1984, it was found that a group of 15–25-year-old women consumed only 75 per cent of the RDA for iron, so many are at risk of deficiency.

Consuming a cup of tea with a meal will reduce the absorption of iron from all non-animal foods in the diet.

Zinc and other trace minerals

Zinc, like iron, is an essential mineral which is required in tiny amounts but also plays an important part in many aspects of the body's normal functioning. It is needed for normal hormone production, certain aspects of brain chemistry, for healthy skin and good resistance to infection. The average daily intake of this mineral for women of child-bearing age in the UK is 7.6 mg per day, which compares favourably with an average recommended daily intake of 5.5 mg. However, like iron and magnesium, a significant percentage, at least five, consume less than the recommended minimum of 4.0 mg per day. Furthermore, the absorption of this mineral is easily upset by alcohol, tea, probably coffee, bran, unleavened breads, chapattis, and many other foods. So a considerable percentage of women may be getting insufficient zinc. Any ill-effects are likely to be slight and subtle, but a deficiency certainly could be a contributing factor to some PMS symptoms.

We are not certain about other trace nutrients. If you are eating a healthy diet with plenty of fruit and vegetables and not smoking or drinking then you are likely to have a good intake of the trace nutrients such as selenium, chromium, copper and manganese. A lack of chromium or selenium may occasionally be relevant for some women with PMS. For example, a lack of chromium does have an influence on the action of insulin and the control of blood sugar. Chromium can enhance the effect of insulin, and correcting a deficiency has been shown to improve blood sugar control. This can be important for some women who are either very overweight or eat a diet very high in sugar and refined foods which are depleted of chromium.

IT'S A POOR SHOW

It seems astonishing to consider that such important nutrients are acknowledged to be in such short supply, and yet not a great deal is being done to reverse the trend. Three out of four of these nutrients do not even have a Recommended Daily Allowance in the UK.

When you read the section on Vitamins and Minerals in Chapter 14, pay particular attention to these four important nutrients, notice what their function is in the body and what happens to us if we don't get them in sufficient quantities. Is it any wonder that our bodies are slowly going to seed when we are not providing them with the essential materials they need in order for them to function properly?

In the Self-Help section, I concentrate on foods that contain a high level of these particular nutrients as well as a few others. I will help you to work out a diet for yourself which will provide you with good amounts of the essential nutrients that you are most likely to be short of.

Other barriers

Not only may we be taking in insufficient amounts of vitamins and minerals, but the value of many of these nutrients is impaired by factors like alcohol, tea, coffee and tobacco.

Another thing to bear in mind which severely lowers the nutritional value of food is the cooking process. For example, boiling a cabbage rids it of about 75 per cent of its vitamin C. Baking or frying food can destroy up to 50 per cent of other vitamins. Commercially frozen vegetables can also be lacking in some nutrients by as much as 47 per cent though usually they are the next best thing to fresh ones, since canning can result in up to 70 per cent of the nutritional content being lost. It appears that processing food does little to enhance our health at the end of the day.

A good example of the effect of processing on nutrient content, is the nutrient content of some of McDonald's foods. I am sorry to keep using them as an example, but at least they are one of the few fast-food manufacturers who have had the nerve to assess the nutrient content of their own products.

By now you no doubt realize that a 'normal healthy diet' is somewhat of a myth. Although it is possible to eat a nutritious diet, you need to be fairly educated on the subject before you can even make a start. Then, as you can see, there are numerous hurdles to be overcome.

Whilst all these facts do seem depressing, there is a light at the end of the tunnel. In the Self-Help section on diet I will be concentrating on which types of foods to buy, and suggesting methods of preparation that will preserve the nutrients in your food.

TIMES DO CHANGE

Is it any wonder women suffer with PMS! One hundred years ago, meat, animal fat and sugar were a much smaller part of our diets than today. The consumption of cereal fibres has also dropped by as much as 90 per cent. These are important factors in relation to PMS, as you will see.

It has become far more difficult to eat a 'normal healthy diet'. However, if you concentrate on avoiding the nutrient-deficient and contaminated foods listed below, you will be making changes for the better in your diet, which will not only help your PMS, but will help you feel healthier all round. There is less you can do to combat the unhealthy effects of the polluted environment, but I make some suggestions below.

The diet of our ancestors. When we examine the diet of our ancestors, we then begin to realize that it is not 'natural' to eat meat in the quantity that the majority of us do today. Evidence shows that diet approximately three million years ago consisted largely of hard seeds, plant fibre, some roots and stems – a diet high in vegetable matter similar to that of the Guinea baboon today.

Animals today are bred to be fat. Modern meat contains some seven times more fat than the wild meat our ancestors ate. Our ancestors' meat also contained five times more of the good polyunsaturated fats than today's meat, which is high in the potentially harmful saturated fats. The ancient diet was also richer in vitamins and minerals and polyunsaturated fats, and many times richer than the modern diet. It was a diet which was largely composed of fresh raw foods.

Antibiotics. Because antibiotics are being so widely used on animals, the conditions that would normally be treated by antibiotics are becoming resistant to them. Apart from being used as a medicine for individual sick animals, they are given to whole herds as a preventive measure, and they are again used for growth promotion.

My advice is to try to use organic or additive-free meat where possible, meat which has not been subjected to drugs, growth promoters or contaminated foods. Organic and additive-free meat is becoming more and more available. Certainly local farms and even supermarkets often keep stocks. If you can find 'clean' meat, it can be included in your diet approximately three times per week. An alternative is to limit one's meat intake to moderate quantities of good-quality lean meat, or to become a vegetarian. It's the fat in the meat that will carry much of the pollutants, so avoid it – and also rely more on fish. When eating chicken, don't eat the skin and don't make the gravy from the fatty part of the juices, pour it off first.

Fat consumption. Britain has the honour of having the highest incidence of heart disease in the world. This was not so in the past, when other countries such as Finland and Australia were way ahead. Something drastic must have happened to change statistics so dramatically.

It seems that the saturated fats increase the level of cholesterol which leaves the bloodstream and settles down in the arteries, resulting in a gradual blockage of those supplying the heart, brain and other organs. This leads to heart attacks, strokes and poor circulation. Smoking accelerates the process.

By 1966 the Australian and US rate of heart disease began to decline, but that was not so for Britain, whose casualties were on the increase.

In other countries such as Finland, for example, who were previously 'top of the coronary pops', a national nutritional education campaign was undertaken. The result now is that they are a much healthier nation with a far lower incidence of heart disease than many other countries.

The sweet facts. Over the past 100 years there has been a 25-fold increase in world sugar production. This is a real change from the days when sugar was an expensive luxury that we locked away for high days and holidays, and was only consumed by the wealthy. Refined sugars simply didn't exist for our ancestors. Their diet consisted mainly of vegetables, fruit, cereals and some wild meat. It wasn't until this century that we developed an addiction to the sweet and sticky sugar family.

We clearly don't need refined sugar. What seems to have been overlooked is that our bodies can change complex carbohydrates and proteins into the sugar they require. Sugar contains no vitamins, no minerals, no protein, no fibre, no starches. It may contain tiny traces of calcium and magnesium if you're lucky, and it certainly provides us with loads of calories (kjs), 'empty calories'.

It is actually a fair skill these days not to consume large amounts of sugar, because it is added to so many foods. What do you think the following have in common? Cheese, biscuits, fruit yogurt, tomato sauce, baked beans, pickled cucumbers, muesli, beefburgers, Worcester sauce, pork sausages, peas, cornflakes and Coca-Cola – well, they can all contain sugar. Coca-Cola contains some eight teaspoonfuls per can.

There are some more nutritious alternatives which I will discuss in the Self-Help section. The food manufacturers are beginning to understand that their consumers are waking up, and the majority actually don't want to be dumped on. For now my advice is to read the labels carefully when you are shopping: I guarantee you will have a few surprises!

Water

Our most important nutrient is water, and sadly it is becoming one of our major sources of pollution. Not only is the water contaminated with lead, aluminium and copper, we now have nitrates to contend with as well. Nitrates are chemicals used in fertilizers to promote crop growth.

Why are nitrates harmful? Well, they go through chemical changes and at the end of the day turn into nitrosamines which are believed to be strong cancer-producing chemicals.

Toxic minerals
Toxic minerals in the form of lead and mercury are in the soil, the air and the water, as well as being present in our food. During this century their levels have been rising rapidly, and at times to a point where our bodies have not been able to cope.

Lead. Lead pollution has been much discussed in the media over the past few years. High lead levels are acknowledged to be linked to low birth weight and low intelligence in children. As a result of extensive research on lead, many countries have removed lead from petrol and are trying to keep lead levels down in cities. However, it is far more difficult to remove it from the water supply as the filtering systems at water purification plants can't always cope with the load.

Helpful tips to avoid the toxins
- Concentrate on eating a nutritious diet, particularly high in zinc, magnesium, calcium and vitamins C and B.

- Take a well-balanced multi-vitamin supplement and some extra vitamin C if you are at particular risk.

- Scrub all fruit and vegetables with a brush to clean off as many toxins as possible, and remove the outer layers of lettuce and cabbage, etc. Don't peel fruit and vegetables unless you don't like the peel – very often the bulk of the nutrients is just under the skin. Use organic vegetables and salad stuff or grow your own where possible, without using chemicals.

- Water filters tend to filter out a good deal of the toxic metals. Water purifiers can be bought in healthfood shops, but they aren't so

105

efficient. Every so often the filter needs replacing – and it's amazing what collects in it. Rather the toxic deposits collect in the filter than your body!

Avoid:

- Spending too much time near busy roads if the local exhaust fumes contain lead (which may be easier said than done).

- Copper and aluminium cookware unless with a non-stick lining.

- Alcohol, as it increases lead absorption.

- Refined foods which give the body little protection against toxins.

- Antacids which contain aluminium salts.

Food additives

Whilst, of course, there are some perfectly harmless substances added to food, the number of potentially harmful additives is significant. Many additives have been shown to cause hyperactivity in children, asthma, eczema, skin rashes and swelling. It's obviously important to be able to differentiate between the safe and not-so-safe additives.

After being bombarded by warnings about additives is it any wonder that some of us have at one time or another avoided all foods containing them? Understandably, 'additive' has become a dirty word in some circles. But it's important to understand that some additives are, in fact, beneficial! For example: beneficial additives include riboflavin – vitamin B2 – and calcium L-Ascorbate which is vitamin C, and the many preservatives which help keep our food from spoiling.

WHICH ADDITIVES ARE SAFE?

Fortunately, there is now no need to remain confused about which additives are safe and which are potentially harmful. Look in Appendix 2 on page 249 for details of booklets and books on additives which will help you to pick out the dangerous additives from the safe ones.

Coffee

Over the last 10 years reports have begun to filter through about the health hazards attached to coffee consumption. Probably one of the reasons why these facts are now coming to light is that increasing amounts of coffee are being consumed. Since 1950 the consumption of coffee in the UK has increased fourfold and according to the US Department of Agriculture, in 1984 10.4 lb (4.6 kg) of coffee were consumed per person in the USA. Many people become quite addicted to it unknowingly, and couldn't give up the habit easily.

We now know that coffee worsens nervous tension, anxiety and insomnia. So obviously, no matter how much we may enjoy it, drinking coffee to excess is not a healthy habit. In fact, coffee contains caffeine which is a mental and physical stimulant. This can be of benefit of course, but even with 2–4 cups per day, adverse effects can be experienced. These include anxiety, restlessness, nervousness, insomnia, rapid pulse, palpitations, shakes and passing increased quantities of water. Regular coffee drinkers not only enjoy the flavour, but in many cases come to rely on the stimulation to get them through the day. If you cannot get going without your first fix of the day, you know what I mean!

Weaning yourself off coffee can sometimes be a fairly traumatic experience. It can sometimes produce symptoms not unlike a drug withdrawal, in particular a severe headache, which may take several days to disappear. However, rest assured they do eventually go completely, as long as you manage to abstain from coffee.

Ways to go about giving up coffee

- Cut down gradually over the space of a week or two.

- Use decaffeinated coffee instead of coffee containing caffeine, but limit yourself to 2–3 cups per day.

- Try alternative drinks like Barleycup or Bambu which you can obtain from healthfood shops.

- If you like filter coffee, you can still use your filter, but with decaffeinated versions or with roasted dandelion root instead of coffee. You can obtain dried roasted dandelion root from good healthfood shops. It may sound a bit way out, but it has a very pleasant malted flavour.

107

Tea

The British are famous for their tea consumption. Tea, like coffee, contains caffeine, about 50 mg per cup, compared to coffee's 100 mg per strong cup. Tea also contains tannin, which inhibits the absorption of zinc and iron in particular. Excess tea produces the same effects as coffee, and you can also experience a withdrawal headache. Tea can also cause constipation.

By drinking a cup of tea with a meal you can cut down the absorption of iron from vegetarian foods to one-third. Whereas, a glass of fresh orange juice with the same meal would increase iron absorption by two times because of its high vitamin C content. Vegetarian and vegan women need their intake of iron to be readily absorbed. Therefore, drinking anything other than small amounts of weak tea may mean they risk becoming iron deficient.

'Herbal teas' don't count as tea as such. It's really a confusing name. Most herbal teas are free of caffeine and tannin and just consist of a collection of herbs. Unlike regular tea, they can be cleansing and relaxing.

Alcohol

Alcohol is causing far greater problems to our society than most of us realize. It is the drug most seriously abused. Young people tend to begin drinking at an earlier age than was the case in previous generations. Public attitudes to drinking have become much more liberal and gradually alcohol has become widely socially accepted, without an appreciation of its adverse effects.

A major factor explaining the rise in alcohol consumption appears to be the decline in the real price of alcohol. It's not alcohol itself that has gone down in price, but the amount of work necessary to earn the cost of a drink.

Before I go any further I must state that I am not addressing alcoholics as such in this section but 'social drinkers'; those who like to have a few drinks, two or three times a week, can be jeopardizing their health. Anything above the national average for women, that is one glass of wine or half a pint of beer or one sherry or vermouth per day, means running some degree of health risk. Men consume on average three times this amount, and are recommended to halve it.

Alcohol in excess destroys body tissue over the years, and can cause or contribute to many diseases. For example, cardiovascular diseases, digestive disorders, inflammation and ulceration of the lining of the digestive tract, liver disease, brain degeneration, miscarriages, damage to unborn children and malnutrition, are some of the conditions associated with the long-term use of alcohol. In particular, certain vitamins and minerals are destroyed or lost from the body, including vitamin B1, thiamin, magnesium, zinc, vitamin B6, pyridoxine, calcium and vitamin D. All of these nutrients are particularly important to PMS sufferers, as you will see in Chapter 14.

As most of these conditions come on gradually, we often don't see the real dangers of alcohol. There is no impact like that of an accident, or the drama of an ambulance arriving to carry you off. But instead, there is a slow process of destruction which conveniently escapes our awareness.

Amongst those PMS sufferers who like a regular drink are those who increase their consumption considerably before their period. If this happens to you, then you will be well aware of the social problems that go with it, such as mood swings and personality changes. When this occurs others around become affected, and relationships may be strained at home and at work. It is a fact that one-third of the divorce petitions cite alcohol as a contributory factor and one-third of child abuse cases are linked to heavy drinking by a parent. Local courtrooms are always having to deal with people who committed offences whilst under the influence of alcohol. Offences that might never have been committed, were it not for that 'one for the road'!

Old habits die hard

The type of food you eat is usually determined by you. However, there are many other factors that influence your 'preferences' through your life. The two main influential factors are:

1   Your parents, who introduce you to your initial diet, based on their preferences and their knowledge about diet.

The chances are that you continue to eat many of the foods introduced to you by your parents through your life. Habit patterns are quite hard to change, and a very important factor, of course, is that you've got to want to change them.

2   The exposure to the media which we all have in the form of advertisements on television, in magazines, billboards, etc. Now, the second factor, the power of persuasion via the media, might be highly desirable – if it was good food that was being promoted. If the media were dedicated to educating the public about a good, wholesome, nutritious diet, a more valuable asset we could not wish for! In reality they are there to persuade

us, on behalf of the food industry, that fast foods, processed foods, or convenience foods, call them what you will, are desirable. They would have us believe that coffee is sexy and that we should switch to cola-based drinks for energy.

Rather than being a help educationally, they are often a great hindrance. Considering how much television we watch, is it any wonder that the hypnotic powers of the media begin to affect many of us, who would otherwise be influenced by common sense and our own good judgement?

Take one positive step at a time

I am sorry to bombard you with so many depressing facts all at once. We the consumers definitely need more information about the food we eat and the environmental factors we are subjected to.

Probably the first step towards reversing the effects of the twentieth century on your body is for you to acknowledge the value of that body if you haven't already done so. After all, we only have one body to last us through a lifetime, so it's important to treat it with respect.

It's up to you how often you expose your body to alcohol, cigarettes, drugs and additives, and how physically fit you keep through exercise. Making one change at a time is better than not changing at all. I will be concentrating on how to go about making changes in the Self-Help section of the book, Part Three.

As for environmental pollution, there are now many worthwhile national and local groups running campaigns to help overcome these problems. You will find a list of these in Part Four. If you are concerned about your local situation, you can always contact the government representative for your area for help and advice.

If you have been neglecting your body to some extent, now may be the time to take stock. Don't expect your doctor to piece you back together again when you have fallen apart through 'environmental wear and nutritional tear'!

It's up to each one of us to look after our bodies to the best of our abilities and to treat them as well as any other of our treasured possessions.

12

MEDICAL TREATMENTS

There are now many different treatments for PMS. The last seven years in particular have seen a flourish of medical publications reporting the effects of a wide variety of different treatment approaches. Their conflicting findings can create more confusion than clarification for both the sufferer and the doctor.

It is understandably hard to imagine why so many different treatments, both hormonal and non-hormonal, can all appear to be effective in treating one condition. Much of the confusion arises because many of the studies conducted have involved only small numbers of women, and have only been performed once, which is really insufficient to prove anything. Also, some of the studies haven't assessed PMS symptoms thoroughly, or explored the possible side-effects of treatment in detail. As a result, we are still in the dark about how effective many of these preparations are in the treatment of PMS.

That said, if we are careful in interpreting these trials, then they can usefully increase our understanding of PMS, and improve the care we can offer to sufferers, especially those with symptoms which may have proved difficult to treat. In an attempt to put the technical findings in perspective, the rest of this chapter is therefore a brief review of the different hormonal and non-hormonal treatments that have ever been tried in PMS. For the technically minded, the relevant references given in the appendix of the book are on page 262.

HORMONAL TREATMENTS FOR PMS

Many of the hormonal treatments that have been put forward as treatments for PMS have been based on the notion that PMS was due to a lack of a particular hormone. Research of the last ten years has, as we have already seen, laid that idea firmly to rest. Even so, some of the more powerful hormonal preparations have been shown to be effective. How could this be? The production of true pre-menstrual symptoms is undoubtedly linked to the normal hormonal cycle. Any treatment that abolishes or suppresses normal hormone production by the ovaries will alter pre-menstrual symptoms for the better, especially if the symptoms are severe to start with. The difficulty with using these types of treatments is that they can produce considerable side-effects, both in the short and long term.

Coming off hormonal preparations may not be easy as they rarely correct the underlying reasons for pre-menstrual symptoms, and the symptoms are likely to return with a vengeance when you stop taking them. Additionally, they are often very expensive. On balance, there seems little justification for using many hormonal products, though we appreciate they may occasionally be useful for individual patients.

PROGESTERONE PREPARATIONS

Progesterone is one of the two main hormones produced by the ovaries. It was once believed that deficiency of this hormone was the cause of PMS, but this is now known not to be the case.

Progesterone pessaries (Cyclogest)

Progesterone, in the form of a pessary inserted into the vagina, has been one of the most popular treatments for PMS. However, seven different scientific studies showed no evidence of any benefit. The latest of these studies by Dr Freeman and colleagues from the University of Pennsylvania involved 168 women. Those who were given progesterone showed no benefit when compared with women who took a placebo (inactive agent). The progesterone which is normally given for 10 to 14 days before the onset of menstruation can no longer be considered as an effective treatment for PMS.

Progesterone tablets

The natural hormone, progesterone, is not active by mouth. Thus for oral preparations synthetic progesterones, known as progestagens, need to be given. Dydrogesterone is one such synthetic progestagen that has been tried in PMS. It has shown modest success in two out of four trials, when compared with placebos. It may also be effective for painful periods and endometriosis, and is particularly suited for women who have PMS and one or both of these conditions together.

Norethisterone is another synthetic progesterone used in the treatment of PMS, though it has not been subjected to much scientific scrutiny. It is effective in the treatment of heavy periods, or delays periods that occur too frequently, and is again best reserved for women who have these problems in addition to PMS.

THE ORAL CONTRACEPTIVE PILL

There are many different types of Pill. Since they were first used in the 1960s, the dosage of oestrogen and progesterone that they contain has fallen dramatically, and with it the risk of side-effects.

The Pill has a variable effect on PMS. In some women it may make it worse, and in others it may improve it; in many it makes little or no difference. It cannot be considered a routine treatment for PMS, but it may be worth trying in women with mild to moderate PMS who require this type of contraception. It should be noted that the Pill can aggravate migraine headaches, and cause an increase in blood pressure in some sensitive women. Women who are overweight, smoke or who have high blood pressure probably should not consider the Pill as an option anyway.

OESTROGEN PREPARATIONS

Oestrogen can come in forms other than the oral contraceptive pill and some of these have been tried in PMS.

Oestrogen implants which are inserted under the skin of the abdomen by a small operation under local anaesthetic have been popularized by Mr John Studd from King's College Hospital, London. He and his colleagues have found them to be highly effective in the treatment of PMS, but they cannot be used long-term because of side-effects, and because the body adapts to the artificially high levels of oestrogen.

Oestrogen given in the form of a patch which slowly releases the hormone into the bloodstream is an elegant and more gentle way of administering this hormone. This may also be an effective treatment for PMS, but is best reserved for women who are approaching the menopause.

When taking oestrogen, you will also need to take progesterone in order to maintain your monthly bleed, unless you have had a hysterectomy.

TESTOSTERONE – THE MALE HORMONE

It may surprise you to know that this hormone, in the form of an implant, has been tried in the treatment of PMS, with some benefit for depressive symptoms but not for physical complaints. It is not a routine treatment.

OTHER HORMONE-RELATED PREPARATIONS

There are a number of other powerful drugs which influence hormone metabolism that have been used in PMS. They can often produce side-effects and are best reserved for special situations.

Danazol:

This drug blocks or interferes with the action of many sex hormones. It can be useful in situations where there is a hormone excess, but anything other than small doses can lead to side-effects, including excessive hair growth, deepening of the voice and other changes. Low doses can be effective in PMS, and are also useful in the treatment of endometriosis, heavy periods and pre-menstrual breast tenderness, if all else fails.

Bromocriptine:

This is another powerful drug which blocks the effect of the hormone, prolactin, from the pituitary gland. It too can be used for pre-menstrual breast tenderness, and in small doses to help PMS, but again it is not suitable for long-term treatment of PMS.

Others

Certain drugs can treat PMS very successfully, by switching off the pituitary gland's stimulus to the ovaries. In this way the ovaries go into 'retirement' and a false menopause is achieved. This abolishes the pre-menstrual symptoms, but not surprisingly replaces them with hot flushes and the risk of osteoporosis. This is really a last-ditch treatment, and has no place for the majority of sufferers.

DRUG TREATMENTS FOR PMS

Just as almost every kind of hormonal treatment has been used in the treatment of PMS, so has almost every type of drug been tried. Many of these treatments have not established themselves as routine therapies.

Diuretics (water tablets)

This in the past has been a popular treatment, particularly in the treatment of pre-menstrual fluid retention and breast tenderness. Many older types of diuretics are effective in the short term, but lead to a loss of the important minerals, magnesium and potassium. Magnesium may be low in some 50 per cent of women with PMS, so further losses would not be desirable. Diuretics are not expected to help mood changes. One type of diuretic, called Spironolactone, has been shown to be moderately helpful, but its manufacturer no longer recommends it for long-term use in young patients.

Most of the symptoms of fluid retention should respond to a diet that is low in sodium (salt) and, if necessary, restricted in calories.

Pain-killers

These can be useful for painful periods, migraine and other headaches that occur just before or with the period. One type of pain-killer, available on prescription only, is Mefenamic acid, which when taken for two weeks before the onset of menstruation may help PMS symptoms. If you experience very painful periods you should ask your doctor for a gynaecological assessment.

Anti-depressants

This type of drug has never been used much in the treatment of PMS. Some of the newer types of anti-depressants may, however, be temporarily helpful in the treatment of severe pre-menstrual depression, especially if you are experiencing suicidal feelings.

Sleeping tablets, sedatives and anti-anxiety drugs

The over-use of these drugs by the medical profession has been of particular concern to many patients over the last 30 years. They have no role in the treatment of PMS, except perhaps occasionally for short-term use in

the treatment of anxiety or insomnia. One type of anti-anxiety drug, Bus-
pirone, has shown some benefit in one small trial in PMS. The method of
assessing its benefit was, however, limited.

All of these types of drugs should be used with great caution, if at all,
and patients should always be given advice about other measures to limit
or control anxiety.

Antibiotics

Extraordinary as it may seem, there has even been a trial of antibiotics in
PMS! This involved giving an old, established antibiotic, Doxycycline, to
a group of women aged 25 to 35 years, 77 per cent of whom also had evidence of vaginal infection. The reduction in PMS symptoms was
accompanied by a clearance of the associated vaginal infection. Other
doctors have related PMS to vaginal infection with *Candida albicans*, a
yeast that causes thrush. The message here is simple. If there is evidence of
vaginal or other infection, then treat it. In doing so one may help PMS as
well.

Other treatments

Many other treatments have been reported as being tried in PMS, including lithium (a drug used to treat certain mental illnesses). Three
studies showed no benefit; Naltrexone (a drug used to counteract the side-
effects of morphine) showed benefit in one small study when given at mid-
cycle; and an anti-allergy treatment showed benefit in one study,
especially in those with an allergic tendency.

Let me finish this chapter with a few conclusions which I hope will help
you make sense of the situation.
1. Do not accept a treatment as proven to be effective unless it has shown
benefit in at least two studies.
2. Powerful hormone and drug treatments probably are effective, but at
the cost of significant short- or long-term side-effects. They are best reserved as a last resort.
3. All treatments can, and should ideally always, be combined with self-
help and nutritional treatments.
4. Many of the above treatments are best suited to those women who have

PMS with associated problems, including period pains, vaginal infection, gynaecological problems, or who are approaching menopause.

5. Many experts now agree that a nutritional approach to PMS is indeed the best first-line treatment. As the nutritional approach is so effective, there will usually be no need to make use of hormonal and drug treatments.

13

NUTRITIONAL
TREATMENTS

Thankfully, in the last few years nutritional treatments for PMS have been taken more seriously. This has come about because of the wider appreciation that many existing medical treatments are not as effective as was once thought and often produce undesirable side-effects, whereas research has shown the value of some nutritional preparations which, as a rule, have no side-effects.

A wide variety of nutritional products have been assessed for PMS, including individual vitamins and minerals, combinations of vitamins and minerals, and evening primrose oil, which contains some specialized fats with vitamin-like qualities. The reason why most of these nutrients were tried in the first place was because of the way in which they are known to influence the function of either hormones or the chemistry of the brain and nervous system, and thus, potentially, the body's metabolism, for the better. But how effective are they?

VITAMIN B6 (PYRIDOXINE)

This has been the most popular nutritional preparation for PMS in years past. Studies conducted in the UK, the Netherlands and Australia have, surprisingly, not found that deficiency of this vitamin is a particular feature of women with PMS, though mild deficiency is quite common in people experiencing anxiety, depression and other mental symptoms. However, it is now known that vitamin B6 influences the action of the hormone oestrogen in the body, as well as being important in the normal function of the nervous system and the processing of protein-rich foods.

At least 13 studies comparing placebo tablets with different doses of vitamin B6, ranging from 50 to 500 mg per day, have been performed. The results are very mixed and a group of Dutch experts who reviewed all of these studies concluded that there was little evidence to support its use. This is perhaps a rather harsh judgement as it may still have a modest beneficial effect for some, and its cheapness means that it should not be discarded completely. If it is to be taken, then a dose of 100 mg per day, every day of the month, is recommended. If it is going to be effective, then there should be improvement within two months. The evidence points to vitamin B6 being more effective if combined with other nutrients.

VITAMIN E

This has long been a popular supplement since it was shown to prevent miscarriages in pregnant rats! Actual deficiency in humans is exceptionally rare, but vitamin E can influence the body's metabolism of fats, which in turn can influence hormone and nervous system chemistry.

Three studies of vitamin E have been performed, all of which have been conducted in the United States. Two of the three studies showed benefit with, curiously, the most effective dosage being 300 to 400 IU (International Units) per day, rather than a higher dose. This may be because different dosages have different effects on female hormones. Certainly it is worth considering; it may help depressive symptoms the most.

MAGNESIUM

Magnesium has, until recently, been a neglected nutrient. For much of this century it has only been considered worthy for use as a laxative. However, it is known to be essential for muscle, nerve and bone function and structure.

The typical diet of developed civilizations can be low in this nutrient if there is over-reliance on convenience foods; an excellent dietary source is green vegetables. This mundane mineral, severe deficiency of which is only rarely encountered, is proving to be one of the most effective bedside treatments in increasing the rate of survival in those suffering from acute heart attack.

It had been suggested by French workers in the 1970s that a mild lack of magnesium might contribute to anxiety and related symptoms. Dr Guy Abraham, from the United States, together with his colleague, Dr Lubran, was the first to show that many, but not all, women with PMS have evidence of a mild deficit of this mineral – a reduced concentration was found in the red blood cells of sufferers when compared with healthy women. This finding has been confirmed in a number of studies including two of our own, and now is perhaps the most consistent abnormal finding in women with PMS.

Unfortunately, only one trial of magnesium alone has been undertaken, and this was by a group of Italian doctors who administered 375 mg per day of this nutrient for two months. There was a significant rise in the level of magnesium and an accompanying fall in the level of pre-menstrual symptoms reported. This important study deserves repetition. Certainly, magnesium is a very promising preparation. It is particularly useful for constipation – it is interesting to note that severe constipation in young women is associated with quite marked hormonal abnormalities.

Magnesium comes in different forms, the most convenient being a tablet. Liquid preparations and crystals of magnesium sulphate (Epsom Salts) are only really useful as laxatives.

MULTI-VITAMINS

Rather than buy them individually, it would seem tempting to use nutritional supplements that combine several nutrients in one preparation. This idea has its merits. It is known that many individual nutrients interact, requiring the presence of their fellows to function properly, and that when someone is deficient in one nutrient, they are likely to be lacking in others as well.

A number of multi-vitamins, usually with minerals, have found their way on to the marketplace in different countries around the world. Virtually all of these preparations have been used without being assessed scientifically. The only preparation of this type that has been subjected to trials published in proper medical journals is Optivite. This preparation is a comprehensive multi-vitamin and mineral supplement that contains substantial amounts of vitamin B6, other vitamins, magnesium and other minerals. It has been the subject of several open or preliminary trials and, more importantly, it has been assessed in four scientific trials where it has been compared with placebo or 'dummy' tablets. The conclusion of these trials from both the United Kingdom and the United States is that it is an effective treatment for PMS when given over three menstrual cycles. The most effective dosage is six tablets a day, every day throughout the menstrual cycle. The effectiveness of this particular supplement may be enhanced by combining it with dietary modification and also exercise. This has very much been our experience at the WNAS in our many years of using this and other nutritional preparations. Interestingly, there is evidence from one American study that Optivite, when combined with dietary changes, does produce a potentially beneficial effect on the metabolism of female sex hormones.

EVENING PRIMROSE OIL

In the 1980s, evening primrose oil became an increasingly popular supplement, and has been the subject of many trials in PMS and other conditions. The particular attraction of EPO is that this oil is rich in an essential fat called gamma-linolenic acid, low levels of which have been recorded in some women with PMS. This interesting fat, and its chemical relatives, does have some influence on hormone metabolism and many aspects of body health. It seems that some individuals may lack the ability to make sufficient amounts of gamma-linolenic acid from other fats in the diet, such as those provided by sunflower and other vegetable oils. Such individuals are particularly likely to benefit from supplements of EPO. This has been the case in the skin condition eczema, where a lack of these fats appears to influence skin quality.

The evidence from scientific trials shows that EPO may be of particular benefit for pre-menstrual breast tenderness, but may not be so helpful for other symptoms. Like Optivite it is best taken when following a healthy diet, as alcohol and a lack of many other nutrients interferes with this delicate area of body metabolism.

The most effective dose of evening primrose oil is 3 to 4 g per day, usually as six to eight 500 mg capsules taken every day through the menstrual cycle. It needs to be taken for four to six cycles, as breast symptoms can be quite stubborn.

The effectiveness of other plant oil preparations, such as blackcurrant seed, starflower oil or borage oil in PMS, is not known as trials have not been conducted. They cannot therefore be recommended.

SIDE-EFFECTS OF NUTRITIONAL PREPARATIONS

No review of the above supplements is complete without mentioning that all of them can produce side-effects, though these are rare and usually much less serious than those that occur with drug-based preparations.

Very high doses of vitamin B6 (pyridoxine) can produce mild nerve damage, causing numbness or tingling in the hands or feet. This has only definitely been described at doses of 500 mg or more per day, as a single nutrient, on a regular basis. Optivite at the effective dosage of six tablets per day provides 300 mg per day of pyridoxine in a slow-release preparation. Nerve damage with this preparation, even at higher doses, has not been reported in any of its numerous trials, nor in the many years of its use, either in the US or the UK.

The main side-effect of magnesium is diarrhoea, which quickly alerts the user to reduce the dose. Magnesium should not be taken by those with poor kidney function, unless under medical supervision, as excessive amounts may accumulate in the body.

Evening primrose oil should not be taken by anyone suffering with epilepsy, as occasionally this condition may be worsened by its use. Again, medical advice should be sought.

All nutritional products may occasionally cause minor symptoms such as nausea, slight abdominal discomfort, diarrhoea or headache. If this occurs they should be stopped for a few days and then tried again at a lower dose. Alternatively, you should obtain some professional advice.

It is unlikely that you will need to take any of these or other nutritional preparations at high or full dosage in the long term. If they prove to be effective, the dose can be reduced, and if not effective, then they should be stopped and a different treatment tried. Some women do find that it is helpful to continue with a modest dose of some supplements, such as vitamin B, Optivite, Femvite (one or two tablets per day) or evening primrose oil (one or two capsules per day) in the longer term. These dosages are safe and reasonable.

We find scientifically based supplements to be a very useful nutritional prop in the short term. Once the symptoms are under control the dosages can be cut back, and very often ex-sufferers can manage with their new diet and exercise alone.

14

NUTRITION AND THE BODY: VITAMINS AND MINERALS, WHAT THEY DO

THE BODY

One thing we have in common is that we all have a body! Our body is nothing more nor less than a highly complicated biochemical machine, the function of which, like any engine, is dependent up on the quality of its food or fuel supply. The body is composed of many different organs and tissues which have important and essential functions and interactions. For example, if you want to move your arm, a tiny electrical message passes from the brain, through the nervous system and down the nerves to the muscles in your arm, which then contract. The degree of stretch or tension in a muscle is relayed, via other nerves, back to the brain, so that the muscle does not over-, or under-stretch in performing the movement that you originally intended.

There are factors that affect the healthy function of nerves, muscles and all other parts of the body. *Firstly, you need to inherit a good and healthy metabolism.* The thousands of chemical processes that take place within each and every cell are mainly determined by the genetic material in the centre of the nucleus of the cell. This genetic material is a master plan or blueprint. It holds the key to which chemical reactions need to take place in order for that cell to function. It determines whether a cell is a muscle cell, nerve cell, skin cell, red blood cell, or any other type of cell. Almost everyone has healthy genes, and thus the possibility for their body to be completely healthy and function efficiently. However, there may be subtle individual variations in metabolism, which determine the strengths and weaknesses of one's physical constitution. This may explain why some people are sensitive to some types of dietary change or nutritional deficiencies, and others are not – why some women may develop Pre-Menstrual Syndrome, and others, despite eating an 'unhealthy' diet, may not.

Secondly, some disease states can lead to the development of PMS.

Finally, and most importantly, there must be a healthy diet, giving an adequate supply of those nutrients necessary for the normal functioning of each individual cell. A lack of any one nutrient leads to changes in the cell's metabolism, which in turn will result in changes in the individual's health.

THE DIET

Many people, when they hear the word diet, think of a weight-reducing or slimming diet. The word diet simply refers to the type of food that a person is eating. Every one of us has a diet of some kind, unless we are starving to death. Certain components of a diet are essential, and many of these terms may be familiar to you. The essential nutrients include proteins, fats, carbohydrates, fibre, water, vitamins, minerals and essential fatty acids. Other factors that are also essential for life include a certain degree of heat and light. First, we should have a brief word about what each of these nutrients does, and why they are essential.

Proteins. These are the building blocks of a body. A protein is in fact a group of smaller building blocks called amino acids, which in turn are composed of individual chemicals. Proteins are found in large quantities in tissue such as muscle, skin and bone. In these tissues protein serves a mainly structural function, contributing to the shape of the body, and its ability to move. Other proteins perform highly specialized functions, such as hormones which influence metabolism, and antibodies which help to fight infection.

We all make our own proteins, mainly in the liver, but to do this, must have a steady supply, from our diet, of amino acids, which are in turn derived from the proteins that we eat. Thus, it is essential for us to eat good-quality proteins, such as fish, eggs, nuts, seeds, wholegrains, peas, beans and lentils and lean additive-free meat. A lack of protein in the diet would lead to loss of muscle function and performance, and to a multitude of changes in the body's metabolism.

Fats. These are providers of energy, and, apart from two essential fats (discussed below), are really not necessary to the body at all. However, every type of protein contains some fat, whether it is an animal or vegetable source of protein. This fat can be burnt by the body to provide energy. The liver and muscle cells in particular can make substantial use of fats in this way. Fats also provide a structural role in forming the walls of each individual cell.

The specialized fat, cholesterol, is used to form the male and female hormones, vitamin D and other important hormones in the body. Our bodies can usually make twice as much cholesterol as we eat. So often a raised level of cholesterol in the blood is caused not by eating too much cholesterol, but a faulty metabolism and a high-fat, high-sugar diet. We certainly do not need to increase our intake of animal fats, as I'm sure you will appreciate after reading the section on fats in Chapter 11, page 103.

Essential fatty acids. These are specialized fats, whose importance is becoming increasingly realized. There are two essential fatty acids, linoleic and linolenic acid. As their names suggest, they are very similar in chemical structure, and both of them are of the polyunsaturated type (i.e. not cholesterol-forming). These perform two main roles. First, they are a structural component of the walls of many cells, and thus contribute to the cellular skeleton of the body. Secondly, these two essential fatty acids can be transformed into a wide variety of different chemical compounds which appear to play a part in hormone function and inflammation. Disturbance in the metabolism of these essential fatty acids has been described in one group of women with PMS. However, this has not been confirmed by a second study. Even so, supplements of evening primrose oil, Efamol, have been shown to be effective in the treatment of pre-menstrual breast tenderness, as well as in the skin condition, eczema. It remains to be seen what role these nutrients play in PMS-causation.

Carbohydrates. Carbohydrates, too, are a source of energy. They can be divided into two categories: simple and complex. Simple ones include glucose, fructose (fruit sugar), sucrose (ordinary or table sugar), and lactose (milk sugar). Glucose and fructose are in fact the simplest sugars, consisting of only one type of sugar each. Sucrose and lactose, on the other hand, contain two different types of sugar joined together, and thus are sometimes known as di-saccharides (two sugars).

Polysaccharides (literally, many sugars), are the 'complex' carbohydrates most usually found in vegetables. These consist of many interlinked sugar sub-units, and in order for them to be used by the body, they must be broken down into simple, single-sugar units by the digestive processes in the gut. Vegetables, wholegrains, nuts and seeds are high in these complex carbohydrates.

The refining of sugar cane and sugar beet to make table sugar, sucrose, results in a loss of some of these complex carbohydrates, and a loss in the vitamins, minerals and fibre present in the original plant. When we eat these carbohydrates they are converted by the digestive processes and the body's metabolism to the simple sugar, glucose, which is a major form of energy in the body. Glucose is essential for the brain, as it can only use this form of fuel. However, one does not have to eat glucose or sucrose, table sugar, in order for the brain and nervous system to have an adequate supply: the liver can make glucose from fats or proteins, as well as from other types of sugars, so while glucose is essential for life, it is a mistake to believe we have to add it to the diet. However, some form of carbohydrate, preferably the complex or unrefined carbohydrates, are necessary for an adequate supply of energy.

Fibre. Fibre is the undigestible carbohydrate residues found in food. Natural or unprocessed foods are usually high in fibre and include wholegrains, nuts, seeds and fruit. Some types of carbohydrate cannot be digested by the human body, and so pass through the stomach and digestive tract to the large bowel. Here, fibre absorbs water and other waste materials, and forms our waste product, faeces. A lack of fibre in the diet often leads to constipation, but it is now realized that fibre has other important functions. Lack of fibre is also associated with such conditions as gallstones, varicose veins, obesity, heart disease and diabetes. Of particular relevance is the fact that fibre binds with cholesterol and hormones that are secreted by the liver into the gut. A high-fibre diet may help in expulsion of excessive quantities of cholesterol and unwanted female sex hormones, but more of this later.

Water. This is of course essential for health. Our bodies are composed of 60–70 per cent water, and many bodily functions are dependent upon water. Water is necessary for vitamins, minerals and other chemicals to dissolve in. The amount of urine produced by the kidneys is largely dependent upon the amount of water consumed. An adequate water intake is necessary to clear waste materials through the kidneys, and to allow normal metabolic processes to take place. Water can sometimes be retained by the body, particularly if the intake of salt (sodium) is high. Both salt and water need to be cleared by the kidneys, and their ability to do this may vary from individual to individual. Women who have suffered with pre-menstrual water retention for years, have managed to overcome the condition by making changes to their diet and taking additional supplements.

VITAMINS

Vitamins are the best-known essential nutrient. Indeed, their name was derived from the term 'vital amines' (a type of chemical). They are named as letters of the alphabet, A, B, C, D, E, and K, and members of the B group are further subdivided by numbers into vitamins B1, 2, 3, 5, 6, 12 and Folic acid. The vitamins themselves, as a whole, are divided into two groups. The water-soluble vitamins include members of the vitamin B complex and vitamin C, and the fat-soluble group includes vitamins A, D, E and K.

Vitamins are vital but only in tiny or trace amounts, unlike proteins, carbohydrates and fats, which are necessary in substantial quantities. These trace amounts of vitamins help modify and control essential cellular reactions. Each vitamin which has particular relevance to the development of pre-menstrual symptoms is described in more detail below.

Vitamin A. This comes in two types : retinol (animal-derived), and beta-carotene (vegetable-derived). Deficiency of vitamin A is very rare indeed, and usually only occurs with a grossly inadequate diet or with severe impairment of digestive function. A lack of vitamin A usually results in an impairment of vision at night, or when in the dark. If deficiencies continue, there are further eye, as well as skin changes.

Recently, a number of studies have demonstrated that either poor intakes of vitamin A, or low blood levels, especially of beta-carotene, are associated with a future increased risk of certain types of cancer, including lung cancer. High intakes of fruit and vegetables rich in vitamin A may thus prove to have a cancer-protective effect.

Vitamin B complex. This is a group of several vitamins with certain things in common. They are all water-soluble, their metabolisms are often inter-related, and they are frequently found together in the same types of foods. Factors that lead to deficiency often, but not always, produce a deficiency of several of the vitamins in this group. Deficiency very often produces mental changes which have many similarities with those of Pre-Menstrual Syndrome.

127

Vitamin B1, Thiamin, is essential for the normal metabolism of sugar. Requirements for this vitamin increase if the diet is high in sugar, refined carbohydrates, and alcohol. Some subtstances which destroy thiamin are found in tea, coffee and raw fish. Good sources of this vitamin are wholegrains, most meats (preferably additive-free or organic) and beans. Any food that is refined is usually quite substantially depleted in thiamin. A lack of thiamin results in anxiety, depression, irritability, changes in behaviour, aggressiveness and loss of memory.

Vitamin B2, Riboflavin, is required for the metabolism of proteins, fats and carbohydrates, particularly in the liver. Deficiency rarely occurs as this vitamin is present in such a wide range of foods, including milk, cheese, meat, fish and some vegetables. Deficiency does not usually produce any mental symptoms. However, vitamin B2 is necessary for the metabolism of vitamin B6 (pyridoxine).

Vitamin B3, Nicotinic Acid or Nicotinamide, is essential for the metabolism of carbohydrates and the release of energy from them. It is found in brown rice, wheatgerm, peanuts and liver. Deficiency rarely occurs unless there is a very poor diet or a high intake of alcohol. In deficiency states, dry scaling and redness appear in light exposed areas, particularly the backs of hands, face, neck and top of the chest. Mental deterioration and diarrhoea are also features, but severe deficiency is very rare. Requirements are between 12 and 15 mg a day. B3 is present in yeast, liver, meat, poultry, legumes, wheat flour and corn. Eggs and milk contain a niacin equivalent called tryptophan.

Vitamin B6 comes in three different varieties: pyridoxine, pyridoxal and pyridoxamine. Pyridoxine is the sort normally used in vitamin supplements, and is also generally used in the treatment of Pre-Menstrual Syndrome. Vitamin B6 requires a supply of vitamin B2 – riboflavin – and magnesium before it is chemically active. Vitamin B6 plays a crucial role in the metabolism of proteins and in the normal metabolism of certain chemicals involved in the brain that control mood and behaviour. Good sources of vitamin B6 include most animal and vegetable proteins, especially fish, egg yolk, wholegrain cereals, nuts and seeds. Bananas, avocados, meat and some green leafy vegetables are also high in this nutrient. A McDonald's Big Mac hamburger contains only 0.02 mg of pyridoxine, which is only 1–2 per cent of that required per day. In fact, it does not contain enough vitamin B6 for the metabolism of the protein contained in the hamburger! Thus a diet containing a significant quantity of such depleted foods, will undoubtedly lead to vitamin B6 deficiency. Other factors which seem to affect it adversely include alcohol and smoking. Deficiency of vitamin B6 produces anxiety, depression, loss of sense of responsibility and insomnia.

Some 15 per cent of women of child-bearing age in the UK have been found to have laboratory evidence of mild vitamin B6 deficiency.

Vitamin B12 and Folic acid. These two types of vitamin B are very important, particularly for the formation of blood and the functioning of nerves. Deficiencies tend to be rare. Vitamin B12 is found almost exclusively in animal produce, especially meat. Long-term vegetarians can be at risk of deficiency unless they take supplements.

Lack of Folic acid can occur from a poor diet, especially if you do not consume plenty of green, leafy vegetables. The name Folic acid comes from foliage, a major source of this important nutrient.

Increased requirements of vitamin B12 and Folic acid occur during pregnancy. Supplements of Folic acid are often given during pregnancy and vitamin B12 should be given to pregnant and breast-feeding mothers if they have been long-term strict vegetarians.

Vitamin C. Almost everyone knows that vitamin C deficiency causes scurvy, and we all think of scurvy as a disease of sailors in the past, and perhaps the extreme deprivation of Victorian times. Indeed, vitamin C deficiency is quite rare but still does occur in some elderly folk. However, in modern times, some people are at risk of having a lower level of vitamin C than is desirable for health. Smoking, in particular, reduces vitamin C levels substantially. The recommended daily intake in this country is only some 40 mg per day, about the amount in an apple.

The increased intake of vitamin C may improve certain aspects of metabolism. In particular, the absorption of iron is helped by the presence of vitamin C in the food. Vitamin C is also necessary for the normal production of sex hormones and the breakdown of excess cholesterol in the body.

Deficiency of vitamin C produces depression, low energy and hypochondria, a condition in which the victim imagines he or she has a variety of different illnesses and complaints. Sometimes, an early sign of vitamin C deficiency is the presence of small pinpoint bruises under the tongue. This seems to be particularly common in smokers.

Vitamin E. Vitamin E is also known as tocopherol, from the Greek words meaning 'child-bearing'. The name is given because rats deprived of vitamin E are unable to bear healthy offspring. Like vitamin C deficiency, vitamin E deficiency is also rare. There are no obvious symptoms or signs of its deficiency, but lack of it is likely to be caused by long-standing digestive problems. Supplements of vitamin E have also been used to treat Pre-Menstrual Syndrome and breast tenderness with some success. It is probable that extra vitamin E is not correcting a deficiency, but improving some aspect of metabolism. The normal daily requirements are in the region of 8–10 mg, which can usually be obtained from dietary sources such as vegetable oils, nuts, green vegetables, eggs and dairy produce.

Like vitamin A, recent evidence has appeared to suggest that low levels of vitamin E in women may be associated with an increased risk of breast cancer in later years. Again, ensuring a good intake of foods rich in such a vitamin may help you achieve good health, not only today, but also for your future tomorrows.

Vitamin D. Vitamin D is necessary for normal healthy bones and teeth. Most of us make adequate vitamin D if our skin is exposed to sunlight. Some can also be provided by the diet as in cod liver oil and dairy produce. Margarine in this country has vitamin D as well as vitamin A added to it. Vitamin D helps the body's absorption of calcium from the diet. In particular, it assists in the normal uptake of calcium into the bones and teeth to make them strong. Too much vitamin D can be toxic, more than 400 international units per day should not be consumed without medical advice.

MINERALS

Minerals are essential components, and may be divided into two types. First there are those minerals which are required in substantial bulk quantities. These include calcium, phosphorus, magnesium, sodium and potassium. They play a large part in the formation of bones and cells. Some other minerals are required in only small amounts and are called trace elements. These include iron, zinc, copper, chromium, selenium and a variety of others. Their main function, like many vitamins, is to help stimulate the complex chemical reactions that take place in the body. A lack of these trace elements, rather like a lack of vitamins, can have a very wide-ranging dire effect upon the body's metabolism. Often the chemical reactions that control energy level and mood, as well as hormone function, can be adversely influenced.

Calcium and Phosphorus. These two minerals often go together, particularly in bones and teeth. It is important to have a good balance of calcium and phosphorus in the diet and the ratio of 2:1 is often recommended. Too much phosphorus will block the absorption of calcium and too much

130

calcium will block the absorption of phosphorus. It is very rare that our diets lack phosphorus, but a lack of calcium is not so uncommon. Good sources of calcium include all dairy products, many nuts, especially Brazils and almonds, bony fish such as sardines, sprats and whitebait, beans, peas, lentils, wholegrains and some green vegetables, especially water-cress. In fact, you do not have to eat dairy produce to get an adequate source of calcium but the rest of your diet must be very well balanced in-deed. Recommended intakes vary between 700 mg and 1300 mg per day. The absorption of calcium is blocked by bran. Bran contains phytic acid, a substance that combines with calcium, preventing its absorption. (Indian chapattis may also have a similar effect.)

Many convenience foods contain phosphates in the form of food addi-tives: soft drinks, including the low-calorie (kj) variety, are notoriously high in phosphate. As a high level interferes with calcium or magnesium balance, these products should be avoided as much as possible.

Magnesium. Magnesium seems to be a particularly important mineral as far as PMS is concerned. Firstly, magnesium, like calcium, is essential for healthy bones as well as nerves and muscles. Lack of magnesium produces poor appetite, nausea, apathy, weakness, tiredness, mood changes and muscle cramps. Good sources of magnesium include most wholefoods, e.g. wholegrains, beans, peas, lentils, nuts, seeds and green vegetables. Water, particularly some bottled waters and tap water from a hard water area, can contain substantial quantities of this mineral, too.

In 1981 Dr Guy Abraham showed that a low level of magnesium was commonly found in women with PMS. Most of the magnesium is inside cells where it is busily involved in chemical reactions. Hence it is the level of magnesium inside the cells – red blood cell magnesium – and not the magnesium in the water compartment of blood that is often low. We re-peated his work on magnesium deficiency in 105 women with PMS and showed that some 45 per cent of women had evidence of magnesium de-ficiency. We don't know precisely how important this deficiency is, but it seems likely that it has an effect on our mental function, the control of the levels of blood sugar and energy, and also the metabolism of some hormones. Unfortunately, there may be no obvious physical signs of mag-nesium deficiency and so it is easily missed.

Like calcium, requirements increase substantially during pregnancy and while breast-feeding, and it is often after a pregnancy and breast-feeding that the worst cases of magnesium deficiency are seen. This may well ex-plain why some women's pre-menstrual problems begin shortly after childbirth. Indeed, magnesium deficiency is also associated with some other problems such as poor contractions of the womb during labour, elevated blood pressure during pregnancy and pre-eclamptic toxaemia. These conditions can be treated by injections of magnesium, an approach often used in the US, but not so much in the UK.

It is important that women with PMS consume a diet rich in magnesium. Sometimes your doctor can arrange for a simple red cell magnesium test to be performed at the local hospital and this may serve as a guide to the use of magnesium supplements.

Sodium and Potassium. These two minerals form an interesting pair. Both sodium and potassium are essential for the normal functioning of almost all cells in the body, particularly nerves and muscles. Since the use of more convenience foods, our diets have had markedly increased levels of sodium. Although table salt and sea salt (both are sodium chloride) represent a substantial source of sodium in our diets, most of the sodium we consume is found in convenience and other tinned, frozen or prepared foods.

Potassium is found mainly in fruit and vegetables, particularly tomatoes, bananas, figs, citrus fruits and almost all green leafy vegetables. Most of the potassium is found inside the cells rather like magnesium, and most of the sodium is found outside the cells. It is the balance of sodium and potassium that is important. This balance has to be maintained: if it is not, then the body may retain water. Too much sodium in the diet is indeed the commonest cause of fluid retention in many women, particularly in the week or so before the start of a period.

Water tablets, known as diuretics, will get rid of this excess fluid retention, but after a while the system gets used to them and the fluid retention returns, sometimes even worse than before. As well as getting rid of the excess water in the body, diuretics have the effect of ridding the body of useful potassium and magnesium, which makes the situation worse.

The answer: reduce sodium intake in the diet by not having salt at the table, not using it in the cooking, and avoiding any salty foods. It is difficult, on the contrary, to consume too much potassium, and problems only arise in patients with kidney disease.

Iron. Iron is one of the most important trace minerals. We all know that iron is necessary for healthy blood and a lack of it results in anaemia. Iron is necessary for the formation of the blood pigment haemoglobin. What is not widely appreciated is that iron is also found in high concentrations in muscles and in the brain. It is necessary for the uptake of energy by muscles as well as for certain aspects of mental function in the normal brain. Iron deficiency is probably the most common deficiency in the world. Women, of course, have increased needs for iron because of their monthly blood-loss due to menstruation. Women who have heavy periods, such as those using the coil, often have increased requirements.

Good sources of iron include wholefoods such as peas, beans, lentils, nuts, seeds and wholegrains, eggs, meat and to a lesser extent fish. The iron from animal sources is easily absorbed, whereas iron from vegetarian sources may not be so well absorbed, particularly if tea and coffee are consumed at the same meal. Vitamin C in the diet may greatly assist the absorption of iron from vegetarian foods.

The features of iron deficiency include fatigue, tiredness, digestive problems, poor quality nails, and recurrent infections, especially thrush. Although 15 per cent of women of child-bearing age are at risk of developing these problems due to iron deficiency, only one-quarter of these women will actually be anaemic. This means that to detect iron deficiency the doctor must not just measure the haemoglobin level but actually measure the level of iron in the blood for a protein associated with iron called ferritin. If you think you are iron deficient *don't* rely upon your own doctor just doing a test to see if you are anaemic. The iron level or ferritin level must be measured and any deficiency treated. Of course, the most sensible thing to do is to eat a well-balanced diet and avoid the factors that can lead to iron-deficiency. It is a good idea not to drink tea or coffee immediately after meals, but only drink it two hours before or after eating.

Any women with continually heavy periods should have this problem looked into. In fact iron deficiency can even be a cause of heavy periods. Now you can see how important a trace mineral can be!

Zinc. Zinc, like iron, affects many different aspects of metabolism, particularly those involved in growth, and resistance to infection. It is necessary for healthy skin, normal hormone production and normal mental function. Adequate quantities can be obtained from wholegrains, nuts, peas, beans, lentils and meat. Like iron, zinc absorption may be blocked by tea and coffee as the tannin from the drink binds with it, preventing its absorption. You know what strong tea can do to the inside of a white teacup – imagine what it does to the inside of your intestines!

Anyone regularly consuming substantial quantities of alcohol, i.e. more than two glasses of wine or a pint of beer per day, is at risk of developing zinc as well as vitamin B deficiencies. Women on the Pill can have lower levels of zinc, as can those who make long-term use of diuretics – water pills. Often a useful clue to a lack of zinc is poor quality skin such as excessively dry or greasy facial skin, particularly at the sides of the nose. Eczema, acne and psoriasis may also suggest a deficiency of this important mineral. Interestingly, the metabolism of zinc and vitamin B6 are closely related, which explains why the skin changes produced by these two deficiencies can have a similar appearance.

Chromium. Chromium is a fascinating trace mineral. Only minute quantities are required: a lifetime's supply of chromium only weighs one-sixth of an ounce (5 g), and the body will only use 1 per cent of that. Yet even this tiny amount of chromium plays a crucial part in the control of blood sugar metabolism. A lack of chromium can lead to poor blood-sugar control, which in turn can lead to fluctuating energy levels and the dreaded sugar cravings. They are a classic feature of some women's pre-menstrual symptoms, as we have seen.

In severe cases of chromium deficiency a diabetes-like state can occur, particularly in older people. Chromium supplements can have a marked effect in this situation, and can also help improve poor blood-sugar control

VITAMINS AND MINERALS – DO YOU LACK THEM?

	Food Sources	What They Do
Vitamin B6	*Meat, fish, nuts, bananas, avocados, wholegrains.*	*Essential in the metabolism of protein and the amino acids that control mood and behaviour. Affects hormone metabolism.*
Vitamin B1 Thiamin	*Meat, fish, nuts, wholegrains and fortified breakfast cereals.*	*Essential in the metabolism of sugar, especially in nerves and muscles.*
Vitamin C Ascorbic acid	*Any fresh fruits and vegetables.*	*Involved in healing, repair of tissues and production of some hormones.*
Iron	*Meat, wholegrains, nuts, eggs and fortified breakfast cereals.*	*Essential to make blood – haemoglobin. Many other tissues need iron for energy reactions.*
Zinc	*Meat, wholegrains, nuts, peas, beans, lentils.*	*Essential for normal growth, mental function, hormone production and resistance to infection.*
Magnesium	*Green vegetables, wholegrains, Brazil and almond nuts, many other non-junk foods.*	*Essential for sugar and energy metabolism, needed for healthy nerves and muscles.*

134

in people who are not diabetics. Eating large quantities of carbohydrates such as table sugar increases the loss of chromium in the urine. There are no outward signs of chromium deficiency, unless you count the presence of old sweet wrappers in the bottom of your handbag! We have seen no end of 'little miracles' as a result of increasing chromium intake: it really is very useful in helping to control the sugar cravings. Eating a sensible diet is the best way to prevent chromium deficiency. Foods which contain a good quantity of chromium are green vegetables, root vegetables, eggs, scallops, shrimps, rye and some fruit.

That ends all you really need to know about vitamins and minerals. It may be useful to summarize this vital information and indicate how you can recognize any deficiencies.

Deficiencies

Who is at Risk	Symptoms	Visible Signs
Women, especially smokers, 'junk-eaters'.	Depression, anxiety, insomnia, loss of responsibility.	Dry/greasy facial skin, cracking at corners of the mouth.
Alcohol consumers, women on the Pill, breast-feeding mothers, high consumers of sugar.	Depression, anxiety, poor appetite, nausea, personality change.	None usually! Heart, nerve and muscle problems if severe.
Smokers particularly.	Lethargy, depression hypochondriasis (imagined illnesses).	Easy bruising, look for small pinpoint bruises under the tongue.
Women who have heavy periods (e.g. coil users), vegetarians, especially if tea or coffee drinkers, women with recurrent thrush.	Fatigue, poor energy, depression, poor digestion, sore tongue, cracking at corners of mouth.	Pale complexion, brittle nails, cracking at corners of mouth.
Vegetarians, especially tea and coffee drinkers, alcohol consumers, long-term users of diuretics – water pills.	Poor mental function, skin problems in general, repeated infections.	Eczema, acne, greasy or dry facial skin.
Women with PMS! (some 50 per cent may be lacking), long-term diuretic users, alcohol consumers.	Nausea, apathy, loss of appetite, depression, mood changes, muscle cramps.	Usually NONE! so easily missed; muscle spasr sometimes.

As a general rule vitamin and mineral deficiencies are caused by a poor diet or the presence in the diet of agents such as alcohol, tea, coffee, cigarettes, poor-quality food, or an excessive consumption of carbohydrates. These increase the need for nutrients from the remaining healthy foods that are consumed. If you have any symptoms or signs of deficiencies which persist despite a healthy diet, or despite taking nutritional supplements for a period of three months, then it is important to consult your medical practitioner. In the Self-Help section on diet, beginning on page 142, more attention will be given to the foods which are high in essential vitamins and minerals and how to have a diet with sufficient quantities of each.

TRIED AND TESTED

The value of the nutritional approach to PMS can be measured in a laboratory. Here are three examples of patients who had 'before' and 'after' laboratory tests. These tests allow us to measure vitamin and mineral levels to verify precise deficiencies which can then be treated.

GERALDINE ELLIS

Geraldine had mainly been troubled by PMS D, and episodes of recurrent thrush. In the past, taking the oral contraceptive pill had aggravated her thrush and worsened her feelings of depression, but stopping the Pill had not stopped the thrush. Similarly, nutritional deficiencies can pre-dispose to thrush, especially a deficiency of iron, and Geraldine was quite severely iron-deficient. The level of iron in her blood was 2 micromols per litre, normal range being 11–29. She was iron-deficient even though she was not anaemic. Iron is necessary, not just for making the blood pigment haemoglobin, but also because it helps to strengthen muscles and improves the digestive system and the ability of cells to fight infection.

Treatment with supplements of iron, multi-vitamins and a further course of anti-fungal treatment to control her thrush resulted in a substantial improvement in Geraldine's pre-menstrual symptoms, clearance of her thrush and correction of the iron deficiency itself. She also had a low level of magnesium in the red cells so required an additional magnesium supplement.

SANDRA PATTERSON

Sandra was a 29-year-old, single girl for whom Pre-Menstrual Syndrome carried a very special significance: on two occasions pre-menstrually she had inadvertently shoplifted. In her pre-menstrual confusion she had forgotten to pay for goods as she left the shop. The mistake was picked up by the store detective before she herself had time to return to the shop and pay for them. The courts put her on probation the first time and Sandra decided she must do something about the Pre-Menstrual Syndrome. She started taking Efamol evening primrose oil, 500 mg capsules, four per day. This controlled her pre-menstrual symptoms extremely well, so well in fact that after a few months she stopped them altogether. Unfortunately, the next month her PMS returned and with it her second shoplifting episode. The court was now beginning to find her story hard to believe.

In fact, the laboratory investigations showed that Sandra had some marked nutritional deficiencies of zinc and vitamin B6. The activity of vitamin B6 in her blood was 46 per cent below an optimum level, the normal range being up to 15 per cent below – this indicated a severe deficiency. Similarly, the level of zinc was also depressed by some 25 per cent. Both zinc and vitamin B6 deficiencies may have influenced mental function and mood. Both play a crucial part in the metabolism of essential fatty acids, a specialized form of which is found in evening primrose oil. Thus it was that evening primrose oil was controlling Sandra's symptoms, without correcting all the underlying nutritional deficiencies. When an appropriate supplement of zinc and vitamin B6 was combined with her evening primrose oil, her pre-menstrual symptoms once again disappeared completely. With a better diet she was able to reduce her need for nutritional supplements. Fortunately the court took a lenient attitude on the second occasion, and she is now well aware of the responsibility she has to look after herself.

REBECCA HARLEY

Rebecca had a long history of Pre-Menstrual Syndrome and low energy levels which showed a significant improvement when her nutritional problems were treated. Investigations showed her to have a very low level of magnesium. The red cell value was 1.5 millimols per litre, normal range being 2–3. Treatment with magnesium supplements, multi-vitamins (especially vitamin B6) and avoiding salt and wheat, made a substantial reduction in her symptoms of PMS H, fluid retention, abdominal bloating, as well as her other symptoms of anxiety, depression and fatigue. However, the fatigue was persistent and she had a rather puffy facial appearance. This suggested that the thyroid gland might be underactive. First tests were normal, but repeat tests a few months later showed that the thyroid was indeed beginning to fail. The pituitary gland, at the base of the brain, normally produces a thyroid stimulation hormone known as TSH. The TSH level had increased to 5.2 micro units per litre, when the normal value should be less than 5. Thus the pituitary gland was producing slightly increased amounts of hormone to try to stimulate the failing thyroid. Treatment with small quantities of thyroid hormone made a dramatic difference to Rebecca's symptoms. Initially, her magnesium level rose to 2.55 millimols per litre, thus showing full correction of the deficiency. An underactive thyroid should always be considered in women with Pre-Menstrual Syndrome, especially PMS H symptoms which do not respond to other treatment. An underactive thyroid may be the underlying cause not only of PMS, but also of heavy periods, a lack of periods, weight gain, decreased energy level, depression, mental sluggishness and dry skin.

RESULTS OF THE WOMEN'S NUTRITIONAL ADVISORY SERVICE PROGRAMME FOR PMS

Over the years the WNAS has conducted a number of studies to assess the value of the WNAS programme. The two most important questions that we have tried to answer are: *How easy or difficult is the programme to follow,* and *How successful is it?*

The first study we conducted was in 1985. Looking at 382 women who were sent a postal programme, we found that at least 245 of them followed the programme either completely or to a reasonable degree. Thus we knew that at least two-thirds of women found the programme acceptable. Further analysis showed that the more closely the programme was followed the more successful the outcome. In those who followed it completely (150 women) 91 per cent of the symptoms marked as severe in the pre-menstrual week reduced to either none, mild or moderate. Overall, 87 per cent of these women felt that they had benefited considerably by three months.

Of the 150 women, 93 were already taking other treatment for their PMS, usually vitamin B6 alone, hormonal treatments, diuretics or anti-depressants. 75 per cent of these 93 women were able to stop all their previous treatment, 16 per cent reduced the dosage and 9 per cent continued unchanged.

In 1988 we looked at a further group of 200 women who had completed all their questionnaires on the postal programme. Again, the degree of improvement depended very much on how closely the programme was followed, particularly for the dietary side of their treatment. 96 per cent of those who had followed the programme reported that they were signifcantly better within the first three months. We also found that women who were overweight lost between eight and 13 pounds, depending on how large they were to start with, without trying! It is now known that even modest weight loss in those who are overweight and have period problems can have a powerful corrective effect on hormonal abnormalities.

In 1990 we conducted a survey of 100 women who began the postal programme and we tried to contact them all so that we had as true a result as possible about the results of the programme. We were able to contact 88 of the 100 women. 69 of them had followed the programme. The reasons why the others had not were: pregnancy, other illnesses such as appendicitis, family stress including divorce and a death in the family, or because the programme was considered too difficult. This last was the case for 10 women. So we knew from this that the programme could be followed by some 70 per cent of women and that the success rate in them was also about 70 per cent. This compared very favourably with the outcome of most drug and hormone trials on PMS.

We tried to learn some lessons from these studies. Firstly, we realized that we had to be as scientific as possible about the supplements, and for many years we have limited our use to those preparations that are scientifically proven to be of value in PMS. Secondly, the diet has to be as easy as possible whilst still being thorough, and this means giving a good number of alternatives. This has become much easier over the years as caffeine-free, salt-free, low-fat foods have appeared on the supermarket shelves. Finally, the better the support from the WNAS the better the degree of improvement.

It was also obvious to us that there will always be some women whom we will be unable to help. As I have said elsewhere, certain medical and gynaecological problems can cause PMS, which will not fully improve until the problems themselves are corrected. We now include a number of questions on our questionnaire to try and identify those who would be well advised to have a gynaecological check.

Our latest analysis has been of those women who attended our clinics in London and Sussex during 1992. These women received detailed, tailor-made advice about their diets with many diet sheets and sample menus, advice about nutritional supplements, some of which were prescribable by their GPs, and advice to exercise. Every effort was made to help women make the necessary changes to their diets. Each woman who attended one of the clinics was either seen again or reported on their progress by telephone. The minimum duration for assessment was two months and most were assessed at three or four months.

Out of a total of 75 women, two women who attended did not actually have PMS but had depression that lasted throughout the month, and they were referred back to their family doctor. The remaining 73 were considered to have moderate to severe PMS and they were all given appropriate advice. Within the first week, two of the women considered that the diet was too difficult for them to follow because of their lifestyles. They both travelled extensively and ate almost all their meals away from home. A further two women could not be contacted because they had moved or were travelling abroad.

This left 69 women, two of whom became pregnant within the first month and were thus excluded from the analysis. (Pregnancy is not a side-effect of the programme!) All of them were asked to complete detailed questionnaires detailing the severity of their symptoms and the degree to which they followed the programme. We found that 97 per cent of the women had complied with the recommendations made, and 82 per cent were significantly better after an average of three to four months. These improved compliance figures almost certainly reflect the greater degree of co-operation that can be achieved in a clinic setting than with a postal programme, and also refinements made to the programme over the years. When we looked further at the relationship between the degree of success and the degree of adherence to the different parts of the programme, again we found that the best improvement was obtained in those who followed the programme most carefully, especially the dietary side.

Only one of the women needed to take a drug, an anti-depressant, because of severe depression in addition to her PMS. Four of the 69 women were also found to have other health problems that had not been previously investigated, and these were: repeated miscarriages, deafness due to a hormone sensitivity, a hormone abnormality related to ovarian cysts, and some unusual food intolerances. All such women needed to be referred to their GP and on to a specialist for further assessment and treatment. Sometimes, therefore, PMS may mask other conditions that require treatment in their own right.

The overall message, I am delighted to say, is that it is a very effective programmme, and that not only does it help to overcome the majority of PMS symptoms, it also provides an education about diet, and a getting-to-know-what-your-body-likes-and-dislikes process, which most of us have missed out on in the past. Energy levels improve, women experience a great sense of wellbeing, and it has a wonderful knock-on effect for the husbands and children, both in dietary and social terms.

15

CHOOSING A NUTRITIONAL PLAN

The Nutritional Approach to PMS is one which involves making dietary and lifestyle changes. It may span a very broad spectrum, in that mild sufferers only need to make a few dietary changes, whilst the moderate and severe sufferers need to follow a more specialized diet and perhaps even change their lifestyle to some degree.

In order to accommodate all PMS sufferers, I have prepared three options for you to choose from:

Option 1 Basic dietary and health recommendations – for mild sufferers.

Option 2 A specialized dietary plan – for moderate sufferers.

Option 3 A tailor-made nutritional programme – for moderate and severe sufferers.

Be guided by the severity of symptoms when making your choice of option, and not the convenience of one regime as opposed to another!

The closer you stick to the recommendations, the better your chances of rapid improvement. It's worth bearing this in mind as you go along, especially if you find it hard going making some of the changes.

OPTION 1 – BASIC DIETARY AND HEALTH RECOMMENDATIONS

1. **Reduce intake of sugar and 'junk' foods.** This includes sugar added to tea and coffee, sweets, cakes, chocolates, biscuits, puddings, jams,

marmalade, soft drinks, ice cream and honey. Consumption of these foods may cause water retention and block the uptake of essential minerals.

2. **Reduce intake of salt, both added during the cooking and at the table.** Also reduce the intake of salty foods, e.g. salted nuts, kippers, bacon, etc. This causes fluid retention and may contribute to other PMS symptoms.

3. **Reduce intake of tea and coffee.** Consume no more than one or two cups of tea and coffee per day. There are many pleasant herbal teas and substitutes for coffee from healthfood shops.

4. **Eat green vegetables or salad daily.** A good helping of either of these should be obtained and eaten every day. Both of these contain important vitamins and minerals useful in the treatment of PMS symptoms.

5. **Limit your intake of dairy products.** They interfere with magnesium absorption, a mineral which is often deficient in PMS sufferers. Restrict yourself to only one serving a day to be safe.

6. **Reduce intake of tobacco and alcohol.** These aggravate some PMS symptoms.

7. **Use good vegetable oils.** A good-quality vegetable oil, such as sunflower or safflower seed oil, should be used for any cooking, or for making salad dressings. Similarly, a sunflower seed margarine should be used rather than butter or other margarine.

8. **Eat plenty of wholefoods.** By 'wholefoods' we mean foods, usually of vegetable origin, which have not been processed or refined, e.g. wholemeal bread and cereals, such as rye, oats, barley and millet. Food such as nuts and seeds are high in vitamins and minerals as too are the important vegetable oils. If eating meat, make sure that it is lean, and eat fish and poultry too. Certain fish, e.g. herring and salmon, contain some essential oils which are helpful in maintaining skin quality and may be of some value in preventing pre-menstrual breast tenderness.

9. **Have regular exercise.** Physical exercise is of proven value in the treatment of pre-menstrual symptoms. Certainly those with a sedentary job, particularly those who do not get into the fresh air, should

take regular physical exercise. Exercise, fresh air and exposure to sunlight are important factors in maintaining health, just as important as ensuring a healthy diet and taking vitamin and mineral supplements.

10. **Take a walk.** In moments of pure desperation or impending aggression, please do immediately take a walk. Get out of the house and change your environment. Walk quietly, taking notice of the things around you. Do this until you feel a bit better.

OPTION 2 – A SPECIALIZED DIETARY PLAN

As well as following the broad dietary recommendations outlined in Option 1 you will need to select a diet that will help your particular symptoms. Once you have worked out which vitamins and minerals you need to concentrate on from the chart below, you can then go on to refer to the food lists and menus that apply to you.

BROAD DIETARY REQUIREMENTS FOR PMS AND OTHER RELATED SYMPTOMS

PMS A – nervous tension, mood swings, irritability and anxiety. Sufferers need high vitamin B6 and magnesium diets.

PMS H – weight gain, swelling of extremities, breast tenderness and abdominal bloating. Sufferers need high vitamin E, vitamin B6 and magnesium diets.

PMS C – headache, craving for sweets, increased appetite, heart pounding, fatigue and dizziness or fainting. Sufferers need high vitamin B6, magnesium and chromium diets.

PMS D – depression, forgetfulness, crying, confusion and insomnia. Sufferers need high vitamin B6, magnesium and vitamin C diets.

Acne/skin problems. A diet high in zinc is needed.

Smokers. Need high vitamin C diets.

Anaemic/heavy periods. Need high iron diets.

144

If, for example, you decide you are suffering with PMS A (Anxiety) and PMS C (Sugar Cravings) you will need to concentrate on a diet high in vitamin B6, magnesium and chromium. You simply refer to the relevant food lists on pages 149-155 when selecting the foods to include in your daily diet. I have also prepared a sample daily menu (see below) plus a sample menu plan for one week. These are designed to give you a guide to balanced menu planning. They are not something you have to follow, but you might like to use them as a starting point.

WHERE TO SHOP

I will be suggesting that you eat plenty of salads, vegetables and fruit. You will have realized from Chapter 11 in Part Two that many of these foods are contaminated with chemicals. Fortunately, most of the large super-markets are now beginning to stock organic produce. Although this is a little more expensive, if you can possibly manage to buy it, you'll be better off. That is, unless you grow your own organic produce, which makes even more sense.

Whilst there are many vegetarian suggestions and recipes included, I have catered for meat- and fish-eaters as well. Again, because of the chemicals and drugs in meat, I would suggest you try to find a butcher who will buy additive-free meat for you from an organic farm.

Changing over to a full range of organic produce is going to take some time. Currently the demands by retailers for organic produce cannot be met. As more and more farmers switch, there will be plenty to go round.

SAMPLE DAILY MENU

Breakfast
Muesli *or* Jordan's Oat Crunchy with a piece of chopped fruit (e.g. a banana, some grapes, berries, etc.)
with milk or yogurt

Followed by:
One or two slices of wholemeal toast *or* Ryvita
with low sugar jam *or* marmalade

Alternatively:
2 scrambled eggs *or* omelette with grilled tomatoes and mushrooms
or boiled or poached eggs
Wholemeal toast or Ryvita and low sugar spreads

Mid-morning snack

See **Snack list** below.

Lunch

Cold meat *or* fresh or tinned fish with salad platter *or* sandwiches
or
Pasta and vegetables
or
Jacket potato with a nutritious filling – for example:
   Tuna and sweetcorn with a little sour cream and black pepper
   Prawns
   Baked beans
   Curried chicken
or
Home-made soup and salad and wholemeal bread or Ryvita

Tea-time snack

See **Snack list** below.

Dinner

Poultry/fish/meat or vegetarian protein served with three portions of
vegetables.
Fresh fruit or a fresh fruit salad
or
choose an appropriate sweet from the dessert section or from the *Beat PMT
Cookbook*

Snack list

Ryvita and fruit spreads *or* peanut butter
Jordan's 'Fruesli' bar *or* Oat Crunchy bars
Scones and low sugar jam
Pasta *or* bean salad

146

Raw vegetables and dips like humus, taramasalata *or* guacomole
Fresh fruit, nuts *or* seeds
Yogurt and fruit

Beverages

Coffee substitutes. Barley Cup, Caro, Bambu, dandelion coffee, chicory, or up to two cups of decaffeinated coffee per day.
Herbal teas. Rooibosch Eleven O'clock tea (with milk). This herbal tea 'look alike', available from healthfood shops, contains a mild, natural muscle relaxant and may help alleviate tension and ease period pains. It is favoured by many of our patients and is definitely worth a try. Other suggestions are bramble, raspberry and ginseng, mixed berry, lemon verbena, fennel and wild strawberry. These days most healthfood shops sell single sachets so that you can 'buy and try' without being saddled with a whole box of tea bags that you absolutely detest.
Cold drinks. Bottled water with or without fruit juice, mineral water, Appletise, Aqua Libra, or Citrus Spring.

A SAMPLE MENU PLAN FOR ONE WEEK

See above for **Beverages.** As your calorie requirements increase by 500 calories per day in the pre-menstrual week, make sure you have a mid-morning and mid-afternoon snack each day of that week in order to keep your blood sugar levels constant. (See **Snack list** on page 178.)

B = Breakfast   L = Lunch   D = Dinner   S = Sweet
Recipes in Chapter 17, page 193.

DAY 1		DAY 2	
B	Orange juice		Apple and celery salad
	Muesli (home-made) with milk	S	Baked pears with raisins
L	Broccoli soup		
	1 slice of wholemeal (wholewheat) bread	B	Fresh grapefruit and orange salad with sunflower seeds
D	Mackerel with herbs (foil-baked)		Toast and dried fruit conserve or sugar-free jam (jelly)
	Brown rice salad	L	Stuffed peppers (bell peppers)

Banana
D Roast chicken
Cabbage
Turnips
Swede (rutabaga) and carrot mix
Sliced fried potatoes
S Slice of date and walnut cake

DAY 3

B Apple juice
Poached egg and toast
L Lentil and vegetable soup
Avocado with crab meat or prawns (shrimps)
Green bean salad
Fresh orange
D Lamb paprika
Brown rice
S Stuffed baked apple

DAY 4

B Wholewheat pancakes (crêpes)
½ quantity dried fruit conserve
½ grapefruit
L Jacket potatoes with tuna
Bulgar (cracked wheat) and nut salad
Orange and cucumber salad
Slice of melon
D Steamed fish with garlic, spring (green) onions and ginger
Stir-fried vegetables
S Rhubarb fool

DAY 5

B Orange juice

Scrambled eggs and tomatoes with toast
L Grilled sardines
1 slice wholemeal (wholewheat) bread
Beanshoot salad
Grapes
2 slices of Ryvita
D Nut roast
Brown rice
Waldorf salad
S Fresh fruit salad

DAY 6

B Grapefruit juice
Yogurt with sliced apple and raisins
L Nutty parsnip soup
Cheese omelette
Red cabbage, apple and bean salad
Plums
D Liver with orange
Leafy green vegetables
Boiled potatoes
Cauliflower and carrots
S Ginger bananas

DAY 7

B Apple juice
Poached haddock
Tomatoes and mushrooms
L Cauliflower and leeks in cheese sauce
Slice of bread
Orange
D Vegetarian goulash
Brown rice
S Fresh fruit salad

NUTRITIONAL CONTENT OF
FOOD PER 100 g (4 oz)

Foods containing vitamin B6

Cereals

	mg
Wholemeal (wholewheat flour)	0.50
Wheat bran	1.38
Soya flour low fat	0.68

Meat

Bacon (lean)	0.45
Gammon (lean)	0.37
Beef forerib (lean only)	0.33
Minced (ground) beef (stewed)	0.30
Lamb breast (roast lean only)	0.22
Veal (roast)	0.32
Chicken (roast meat only)	0.26
Duck (roast meat only)	0.25
Turkey (roast meat only)	0.32
Liver (stewed)	0.64

Fish

Cod (baked)	0.38
Cod (grilled)	0.41
Salmon (steamed)	0.83
Plaice (steamed)	0.47
Herring (grilled)	0.57
Kipper (baked)	0.57
Mackerel (fried)	0.84

Fruit

Bananas (raw)	0.51
Apricots dried (raw)	0.17
Prunes dried (raw)	0.24
Raisins dried	0.30

Vegetables and pulses

	mg
Butter (lima) beans (raw)	0.58
Haricot beans (raw)	0.56
Mung beans (raw)	0.50
Red kidney beans (raw)	0.44
Broccoli tops (boiled)	0.13
Brussels sprouts (boiled)	0.17
Cabbage red (raw)	0.21
Cauliflower (boiled)	0.12
Avocado pear	0.42
Leeks (boiled)	0.15
Potatoes (boiled and baked)	0.18

Nuts

Hazelnuts	0.55
Peanuts	0.50
Walnuts	0.73

Other

Tomato purée (paste)	0.63
Bovril (Miso)	0.53
Marmite (Miso)	1.3

Foods containing magnesium

Cereals

Wheat bran	520
Wholemeal (wholewheat) flour	140
Oatmeal (raw)	110
Porridge (rolled) oats	30
Soya flour (low fat)	290
Wholemeal (wholewheat) bread	230
Muesli	100

149

Dairy	mg
Dried skimmed (skim) milk	117
Fresh whole milk	12

Meat	mg
Beef (lean cooked)	11
Lamb (lean cooked)	12
Chicken meat (roast)	24
Sheep's heart (roast)	35

Fish	mg
Cod (baked)	26
Herring (grilled)	32
Kipper (baked)	48
Pilchards (canned)	39
Salmon (steamed)	29
Sardines (canned in oil)	52
Winkles (boiled)	360
Crab (boiled)	48

Fruit (raw)	mg
Pineapple (fresh)	17
Apricots (fresh)	12
Apricots (dried)	65
Bananas	42
Blackberries	30
Dates (dried)	59
Figs (dried)	92
Raisins (dried)	42
Passion-fruit	39
Sultanas (golden raisins)	35
Prunes (dried)	27

Nuts	mg
Almonds	260
Brazil	410
Walnuts	130
Peanuts	180

Vegetables and Pulses	mg
Butter (lima) beans (boiled)	33
Haricot beans (boiled)	45
Mung beans (raw)	170
Chick peas (dahl) (cooked)	67
Spinach (boiled)	59
Sweetcorn (boiled)	45
Potatoes baked (with skins)	24
Avocado pear	29

Beverages/drinks	mg
Infusion sachet	6
Indian tea	250

Other	mg
Black treacle (molasses)	140

Foods containing zinc

Cereals	
Wheat bran	16.2
Wholemeal (wholewheat) flour	3.0

Dairy	
Milk whole	0.35
Dried whole milk	3.2
Dried skimmed (skim) milk	4.1
Cheddar cheese	4.0
Parmesan cheese	4.0
Yogurt	0.60

Eggs	
Egg (boiled)	1.5
Egg yolk (raw)	3.6
Egg (poached)	1.5

Meat

	mg
Bacon (cooked)	0.8
Beef (lean roast)	6.8
Lamb (cooked)	1.4
Lamb chops (lean only grilled)	4.1
Pork (grilled lean only)	3.5
Chicken (roast meat)	1.4
Turkey (roast meat)	2.4
Liver (fried)	6.0

Nuts

Almonds	3.1
Brazils	4.2
Hazelnuts	2.4
Peanuts	3.0
Walnuts	3.0

Fish

Cod (baked)	0.5
Plaice (fried)	0.7
Herring (grilled)	0.5
Mackerel (fried)	0.5
Salmon (canned)	0.9
Sardines (canned in oil)	3.0
Tuna (canned)	0.8
Crab (boiled)	5.5
Prawns (shrimps) (boiled)	2.1
Oysters (raw)	45.0
Mussels (boiled)	2.1

Vegetables and Pulses

Butter (lima) beans (boiled)	1.0
Savoy cabbage (boiled)	0.2
Cabbage red (raw)	0.3
Lentils split (boiled)	1.0
Peas fresh (boiled)	0.5
Lettuce	0.2
Spinach (boiled)	0.4
Sweetcorn (boiled)	1.0

Other

	mg
Ginger (ground)	6.8

Foods containing iron

Cereals

Bemax (wheat germ)	10.0
Wheat bran	12.9
Rice	0.5

Meat

Beef (lean cooked)	1.4
Rumpsteak (boneless sirloin) (lean only grilled)	3.5
Lamb (lean roast)	2.5
Lamb kidney	12.0
Pork lean (grilled)	1.2
Pig liver (stewed)	17.0
Veal	1.2
Chicken (dark meat)	1.0
Chicken (liver fried)	9.1
Bovril (Miso)	14.0

Eggs

Egg whole (boiled)	2.0
Egg yolk (raw)	6.1

Fish

Mackerel (fried)	1.2
Sardines (canned in oil)	2.9
Trout (steamed)	1.0
Crab (boiled)	1.3
Prawns (shrimps) (boiled)	1.1
Cockles (boiled)	26.0
Mussels (boiled)	7.7
Oysters (raw)	6.0
Scallops (steamed)	3.0

Nuts	mg
Almonds	4.2
Brazils	2.8
Coconut (fresh)	2.1

Dairy	
Cheddar cheese	0.40

Vegetables and Pulses

	mg
Haricot beans (boiled)	2.5
Mung beans (raw)	8.0
Red kidney beans	6.7
Avocado pear	1.5
Lentils (boiled)	2.4
Butter (lima) beans (boiled)	1.7
Parsley	8.0
Spring greens (cabbage) (boiled)	1.3
Leeks (boiled)	2.0

Fruit

Apricots	0.4
Bananas	0.4
Blackberries	0.9
Dates (dried)	1.6
Figs (dried)	4.2
Sultanas (golden raisins) (dried)	1.8
Prunes (dried)	2.9
Raisins (dried)	1.6
Strawberries	0.7

Foods containing vitamin C

Dairy	
Milk fresh whole	1.5
Natural yoghurt	0.4

Vegetables	mg
Asparagus (boiled)	20
Runner beans (boiled)	5
Broad (sava) beans (boiled)	15
Broccoli tops (boiled)	34
Brussels sprouts (boiled)	40
Cabbage red (raw)	55
Radishes	25
Spinach (boiled)	25
Watercress	60
Cauliflower (boiled)	20
Spring greens (cabbage)	30
Avocado pear	15
Leeks (boiled)	15
Lettuce	15
Mustard and cress	40
Onions (raw)	10
Spring onions (scallions) (raw)	25
Parsley	150
Parsnips (boiled)	10
Peas fresh (boiled)	15
Peppers (bell peppers) green (boiled)	60
Potatoes (baked)	5-16

Meat	
Lamb kidney	9.0

Fruit (raw unless otherwise stated)

Apples	10
Apples (baked with sugar)	14
Apricots (fresh)	7
Banana	10
Blackberries	20
Blackcurrants	200
Gooseberries green (stewed)	31
Grapes (white)	4
Grapefruit	40
Guavas (canned)	180

Fruit (continued)

	mg
Lemons (whole)	80
Lychees	40
Oranges	50
Orange juice (fresh)	50
Peaches (fresh)	8
Pears (eating)	3
Pineapple (fresh)	25
Plums	3
Raspberries	25
Rhubarb (stewed)	8
Strawberries	60
Coconut (fresh)	2
Grapefruit juice (unsweetened)	28

Note: Nuts generally have only a trace of vitamin C

Foods containing vitamin E

Oils

Cod liver oil	20.0
Sunflower seed oil	48.7
Peanut oil	13.0
Olive oil	5.1

Meat

Lamb (cooked)	0.18
Lamb kidney	0.41
Pork (cooked)	0.12
Chicken (roast meat only)	0.11

Eggs

Egg (boiled/poached)	1.6

Fish

Cod (baked)	0.59
Halibut (grilled)	0.90
Herring (grilled)	0.30

	mg
Mussels (boiled)	1.2
Salmon (canned)	1.5
Tuna (canned in oil)	6.3

Nuts

Almonds	20.0
Brazils	6.5
Hazelnuts	21.0
Peanuts	8.1

Fruit

Blackberries (raw)	3.5
Blackcurrants	1.0

Vegetables

Asparagus (boiled)	2.5
Broccoli tops (boiled)	1.1
Brussels sprouts (boiled)	0.9
Parsley	1.8
Spinach (boiled)	2.0
Avocado	3.2

Foods containing calcium

Cereals

Brown flour	150
Oatmeal (uncooked)	55
Soya flour	210
Wholemeal (wholewheat) bread	23
Brown bread	100
Muesli	200

Fish

Haddock (fried)	110
Pilchards (canned in tomato sauce)	300
Sardines (canned in oil)	550

Fish (continued)

	mg
Sprats (fried)	710
Tuna (canned in oil)	7
Shrimps (boiled)	320
Whitebait (fried)	860
Salmon (canned)	93
Kipper (baked)	65
Plaice (steamed)	38

Fruit

	mg
Apricots (dried)	92
Blackberries (raw)	63
Figs (dried)	280
Lemons (whole)	110
Rhubarb (stewed)	93
Tangerines	42

Dairy

Milk	120
Milk dried (skimmed/skim)	1190
Cheddar cheese	800
Parmesan cheese	1220
Cottage cheese (ricotta)	800
Yogurt (natural)	180

Vegetables and Pulses

Carrots (raw)	48
Celery (raw)	52
Parsley (raw)	330
Spinach (boiled)	600
Watercress	220
Turnips (boiled)	55
French beans (boiled)	39
Haricot beans (boiled)	65
Broccoli tops (boiled)	61
Spring greens (cabbage) (boiled)	86

Nuts

	mg
Almonds	250
Brazil nuts	180
Peanuts	61

Foods containing chromium

The following foods are known to contain chromium.

Meat

Calf liver	55
Chicken	15
Lamb chops	12
Pork chops	10

Eggs

Hens' eggs	16

Fish

Scallops	11
Shrimps	7

Cereals

Rye bread	30

Dairy

Milk	1
Butter	13

Fruit

Apple	14
Banana	10
Orange	5

Fruit (continued)

	mg
Strawberries	3

Vegetables

	mg
Cabbage	4
Carrots	9
Fresh chilli	30
Green beans	4
Green (bell) peppers	19

	mg
Lettuce	7
Mushrooms	4
Parsnips	13
Potatoes	24
Spinach	10

Other

	mg
Brewer's yeast	112

Foods containing polyunsatured fats

Certain fish contain essential oils, similar to those found in vegetables. These oils are helpful in maintaining skin quality and may also be of value in preventing pre-menstrual breast tenderness.

Herring
Mackerel
Pilchard
Salmon
Sardines
Sprats
Whitebait

How to begin

In the next chapter 'A tailor-made nutritional programme' you will find details about charting your symptoms and keeping daily diaries as a record of your progress. I suggest you do the following:

Complete a chart before you begin so that you have a clear picture of your symptoms.

- Follow the specialized diet for a period of three months.

- Keep daily diaries of all your symptoms. These are provided on page 256 at the end of the book.

- Complete another chart after three months. This can then be compared with your first chart to measure your progress.

155

16

A TAILOR-MADE NUTRITIONAL PROGRAMME – OPTION 3

The tailor-made nutritional programme is designed to help overcome severe symptoms. Having said that, I feel I should also point out that it is a tough programme, and if your symptoms are extremely severe, you may need help initially. If you can't manage to work out your own programme or you feel you need support, you can contact us at the Women's Nutritional Advisory Service.

Before getting too enthusiastic, it's important to understand that 'The Nutritional Programme' involves quite a bit of work. It's not a magic pill or potion that works overnight in your sleep, but an organized regime that requires a substantial amount of will-power to start with.

At the Women's Nutritional Advisory Service we try to work out the best programme for each individual, according to their symptoms and their existing lifestyle. A *realistic* regime stands a good chance of being followed, whereas an idealistic programme that would work wonders in theory is useless if left in a drawer and forgotten about because it's just too difficult to face or follow.

In order to work out each individual's programme, we need a fair amount of information. As I don't have your chart in front of me I can't work out your programme in the usual way. What I *can* do is to set you a series of questions, and then explain to you, according to your answers, how you go about working out your own programme. I will be unveiling some 'trade secrets' in the course of this section of the book, and hopefully most aspects of the Pre-Menstrual Syndrome will have been covered.

YOUR PERSONAL NUTRITIONAL PROGRAMME

This programme is designed to help moderate and severe sufferers over their symptoms. If you feel your symptoms fit into the definition of moderate or severe on page 160, you would be best advised to follow this more specialized tailor-made nutritional plan. Make a start in completing the chart and the diary provided on pages 159 and 257. Once you are satisfied with your answers, usually after one full cycle, you can begin compiling your own programme.

If you prefer to begin immediately without waiting for the forms to be completed, then I suggest you follow Option 2 – A Specialized Dietary Plan on page 144. Once your precise programme has been formulated you can implement the additional recommendations and make any changes that are needed.

To avoid confusion, remember that recommendations according to your symptoms should be followed in the long term for best results, rather than continuing to follow the general recommendations made in previous chapters. The reason I make this point is that you may find the two sets of instructions conflict in some areas. An example is that the general recommendations suggest eating plenty of whole grains. However we often find that severe symptoms may be aggravated by certain grains and we may therefore suggest that these are omitted from the diet for a specific period of time in some cases. I have covered this in much fuller detail in the section on food allergies on page 171.

A STEP-BY-STEP GUIDE
TO WORK OUT YOUR OWN PROGRAMME

STEP ONE – HOW TO CHART YOUR SYMPTOMS

Begin by completing the first Pre-Menstrual Syndrome Chart on page 159. This should ideally be completed in two parts.

The left-hand column deals with how you feel normally when you are *not* pre-menstrual. *This column should be completed three days after your period has started or when you feel at your best.*

The right-hand column deals with how you feel pre-menstrually when your symptoms are at their worst. *This column should be completed two days before your period is due or when you feel at your worst.*

ANITA WALKER

SYMPTOMS

Symptom	After: None	Mild	Moderate	Severe	Before: None	Mild	Moderate	Severe
PMS - A								
Nervous Tension	✓							✓
Mood Swings	✓							✓
Irritability	✓							✓
Anxiety	✓							✓
PMS - H								
*Weight Gain	✓							✓
Swelling of Extremities			✓					
Breast Tenderness	✓							✓
Abdominal Bloating		✓						✓
PMS - C								
Headache	✓						✓	
Craving for Sweets	✓							✓
Increased Appetite	✓							✓
Heart Pounding	✓				✓			
Fatigue	✓							✓
Dizziness or Fainting	✓				✓			
PMS - D								
Depression	✓							✓
Forgetfulness	✓							✓
Crying	✓						✓	
Confusion	✓							✓
Insomnia	✓							✓
OTHER SYMPTOMS								
Loss of Sexual Interest	✓					✓		
Disorientation	✓							✓
Clumsiness	✓							✓
Tremors/Shakes	✓							✓
Thoughts of Suicide	✓							✓
Agoraphobia	✓							
Increased Physical Activity	✓				✓			
Heavy/Aching Legs	✓							✓
Generalized Aches	✓							✓
Bad Breath	✓							✓
Sensitivity to Music/Light	✓				✓			
Excessive Thirst	✓							✓

Do you have any other PRE-MENSTRUAL SYMPTOMS not listed above?

1. _____
2. _____
3. _____
4. _____
*5. How much weight do you gain before your period? 7–10lbs

158

SYMPTOMS

SYMPTOMS	WEEK AFTER PERIOD (Fill in 3 days after period)				WEEK BEFORE PERIOD (Fill in 2-3 days before period)			
	None	Mild	Moderate	Severe	None	Mild	Moderate	Severe
PMS - A								
Nervous Tension								
Mood Swings								
Irritability								
Anxiety								
PMS - H								
*Weight Gain								
Swelling of Extremities								
Breast Tenderness								
Abdominal Bloating								
PMS - C								
Headache								
Craving for Sweets								
Increased Appetite								
Heart Pounding								
Fatigue								
Dizziness or Fainting								
PMS - D								
Depression								
Forgetfulness								
Crying								
Confusion								
Insomnia								
OTHER SYMPTOMS								
Loss of Sexual Interest								
Disorientation								
Clumsiness								
Tremors/Shakes								
Thoughts of Suicide								
Agoraphobia								
Increased Physical Activity								
Heavy/Aching Legs								
Generalized Aches								
Bad Breath								
Sensitivity to Music/Light								
Excessive Thirst								

Do you have any other PRE-MENSTRUAL SYMPTOMS not listed above?

1. _____

2. _____

3. _____

4. _____

*5.   How much weight do you gain before your period? _____

In order to work out your score, you must place a tick by each symptom in both columns. On page 158 is an example of a completed chart. You can see how the symptoms become far more severe pre-menstrually (on the right-hand side of the chart).

Severity of symptoms

You will notice that on the chart you are asked to assess whether your symptoms are mild, moderate or severe. Each of these categories has a numerical score as follows:

0 = None.
1 = Mild.
2 = Moderate.
3 = Severe.

Mild, moderate and severe defined

(1) Mild   Means that symptoms are present but they do not interfere with your activities. You feel all right, but are aware that some physical and emotional changes are taking place as your period approaches.

(2) Moderate Means that symptoms are present and they do interfere with some activities, but they are not disabling. You feel well below par and maybe even cancel arrangements. The family would be aware your period is on its way, maybe even before you are.

(3) Severe Means that symptoms are not only present, they interfere with all activities. They are severely disabling and it's likely that life would be pretty hard to cope with until the symptoms pass.

Using Anita's first chart on page 158 as an example, let's go through it section by section so that you can understand how it works.

PMS A, H, C and D

PMS A – Anxiety. In order to 'qualify' for PMS A your score must be 4 or above for this section. To get your final score you subtract the score for the week after your period from the score for the week before your period.

Anita scored 0 after her period and 12 pre-menstrually. Therefore, her overall score is 12, so she certainly does qualify for PMS A.

The reason for subtracting one score from another in this fashion is to attempt to get the *actual* pre-menstrual score. For example, if you have moderate regular headaches all month and they become severe pre-menstrually your real pre-menstrual headache score is only 1, as this symptom only moved from mild to moderate. Compare this to another person who usually has no headaches, but has severe pre-menstrual headaches: the pre-menstrual headache score would be 3 here.

Not to subtract the usual situation for the rest of your cycle from the pre-menstrual situation would create a false picture.

This method of scoring applies to all four categories.

PMS H – Hydration. For PMS H you also need a score of 4 to qualify. Anita scored 3 after her period and 10 before her period, giving her a total score of 7. She therefore qualifies.

PMS C – Sugar craving. For PMS C there are six symptoms. You will need an overall score of 6 to qualify. Anita scored 0 after her period and a score of 11 before her period. Her overall score was therefore 11.

PMS D – Depression. And finally for PMS D, a score of 5 is necessary as there are five symptoms listed in this category. Anita scored 0 after her period and 14 pre-menstrually. Her total score here was 14. She qualified with honours!

Once you have completed your chart you can go on to work out your scores using this example.

Each category has been dealt with separately. You may find that only one of the four categories applies to you. However, it is perfectly possible to be suffering from several categories, or in fact all four.

Now fill in your first chart and see how you fare.

You will notice an additional section on the chart. This is made up of other symptoms which have been reported repeatedly by patients.

Is it really pre-menstrual?

The best way to assess your symptoms in order to confirm that they are pre-menstrual is to keep daily diaries as I mentioned previously. After two or three months you will see a definite pattern emerging which will serve to confirm the diagnosis of PMS. Two diaries have been provided for this purpose beginning on page 258. Please feel free to photocopy the diaries if you wish.

If, after three months, it seems that your scores are low and your symptoms seem to be persisting all month rather than pre-menstrually, then it would be best to have a full medical consultation and physical examination to determine whether there is some other problem.

Diaries

It is not only a good idea, but essential that you keep daily diaries. In fact, some doctors feel that it is necessary to keep a diary for three months in order to confirm the diagnosis of PMS. There are several reasons for this:

- To keep a check on your symptoms.

- To confirm that you have PMS.

- To show a pattern of when the symptoms occur each month.

- To have as a record so that you can judge whether improvement is occurring, without having to rely on your memory.

The form we use is called the Menstrual Symptomatology Diary (MSD), and was designed by Dr Abraham to enable sufferers to keep an ongoing record of their symptoms. The diary should be filled in at the end of each day, throughout the cycle. There are a few things to remember when you do this:

The first day of your cycle is the day your period begins. Whether your period comes every 22 days or 32 days is irrelevant here. The day bleeding begins, you start a new diary calling this *Day 1*.

There is an example of a completed diary opposite.

Now you should start filling in the diary and continue to fill it in at the end of each day.

After a few months you should see a very definite pattern emerging. The most likely pattern is for you to experience few symptoms once your period has arrived until at least ovulation, that is, mid cycle. So you will fill in only noughts in the diary. If you have any symptoms at ovulation, indicate them vertically, according to their severity. As your period approaches, the number you fill in will probably get higher, at least for the symptoms that bother you.

MENSTRUAL SYMPTOMATOLOGY DIARY

Month: January

GRADING OF MENSES

0–none	3–heavy
1–slight	4–heavy and
2–moderate	clots

GRADING OF SYMPTOMS (COMPLAINTS)

0–none
1–mild-present but does not interfere with activities
2–moderate-present and interferes with activities but not disabling
3–severe-disabling. Unable to function.

Day of cycle	1	2	3	4	5	6	7	8	9	10	11	12	13	14	15	16	17	18	19	20	21	22	23	24	25	26	27	28	29
Date	13	14	15	16	17	18	19	20	21	22	23	24	25	26	27	28	29	30	31	1	2	3	4	5	6	7	8	9	10
Period	1	2	3	3	2	1	0	0	0	0	0	0	0	0	0	0	0	0	0	0	0	0	0	0	0	0	0	0	0

PMS - A

	1	2	3	4	5	6	7	8	9	10	11	12	13	14	15	16	17	18	19	20	21	22	23	24	25	26	27	28	29
Nervous tension	1	0	0	0	0	0	0	0	0	0	0	0	0	0	0	0	0	0	0	1	0	1	1	2	2	3	3	3	2
Mood swings	0	0	0	0	0	0	0	0	0	0	0	0	0	0	0	0	0	0	1	2	1	2	2	3	2	3	2	2	3
Irritability	0	0	0	0	0	0	0	0	0	0	0	0	0	0	0	0	0	0	0	1	1	2	2	2	2	2	3	3	3
Anxiety	0	0	0	0	0	0	0	0	0	0	0	0	0	0	0	0	0	1	1	0	0	2	3	3	2	2	2	3	2

PMS - H

	1	2	3	4	5	6	7	8	9	10	11	12	13	14	15	16	17	18	19	20	21	22	23	24	25	26	27	28	29
Weight gain	0	0	0	0	0	0	0	0	0	0	0	0	0	0	0	0	0	0	1	1	1	2	2	2	3	2	2	3	3
Swelling of extemities	0	0	0	0	0	0	0	0	0	0	0	0	0	0	0	0	0	0	0	1	1	1	1	2	2	2	2	2	2
Breast tenderness	0	0	0	0	0	0	0	0	0	0	0	0	0	0	0	0	0	0	1	1	1	1	2	2	2	2	2	2	2
Abdominal bloating	1	0	0	0	0	0	0	0	0	0	0	0	0	0	0	0	0	1	1	2	2	2	1	2	1	1	2	2	2

PMS - C

	1	2	3	4	5	6	7	8	9	10	11	12	13	14	15	16	17	18	19	20	21	22	23	24	25	26	27	28	29
Headache	0	0	0	1	0	0	0	0	0	0	0	0	0	0	0	0	0	0	0	0	0	0	0	0	0	2	0	0	1
Craving for sweets	0	0	0	0	0	0	0	0	0	0	0	0	0	0	0	0	1	2	2	0	1	2	3	3	3	2	1	2	2
Increased appetite	0	0	0	0	0	0	0	0	0	0	0	0	0	0	0	0	0	3	2	2	1	0	0	2	2	2	2	2	2
Heart pounding	0	0	0	0	0	0	0	0	0	0	0	0	0	0	0	0	0	0	0	0	0	0	0	0	0	0	0	0	0
Fatigue	1	1	2	1	0	0	0	0	0	0	0	0	0	0	0	0	0	0	0	2	2	3	3	3	3	3	3	3	3
Dizziness or faintness	1	0	0	0	0	0	0	0	0	0	0	0	0	0	0	0	0	0	0	0	0	0	0	0	0	0	0	0	0

PMS - D

	1	2	3	4	5	6	7	8	9	10	11	12	13	14	15	16	17	18	19	20	21	22	23	24	25	26	27	28	29
Depression	1	0	0	0	0	0	0	0	0	0	0	0	0	0	0	0	0	0	1	1	1	2	2	2	3	3	3	3	3
Forgetfulness	0	0	0	0	0	0	0	0	0	0	0	0	0	0	0	0	1	0	3	2	3	3	3	3	3	2	2	3	3
Crying	0	0	0	0	0	0	0	0	0	0	0	0	0	0	0	0	1	0	1	2	1	2	3	3	3	2	3	3	3
Confusion	1	0	0	0	0	0	0	0	0	0	0	0	0	0	0	0	0	1	2	2	2	2	2	3	3	2	2	2	2
Insomnia	1	1	0	0	0	0	0	0	0	0	0	0	0	0	0	0	0	1	1	1	1	1	2	2	2	1	3	3	3

PAIN

Cramps (low abdominal)																													
Backache																													
General aches/pains																													

NOTES:

STEP TWO – PLANNING YOUR DIET

Making changes

Unfortunately there seems to be some truth in the saying 'old habits die hard'. If you set out bearing this in mind you won't get disillusioned along the way. Following the programme usually involves making quite a few changes in both diet and lifestyle. To be realistic, it does take a while to adjust fully. The first month is usually the most rocky. The new routine may cause a bit of confusion here and there at first and a few surprises along the way. If it seems difficult, remember, it is important to persist until you are out of the woods.

Forewarned is forearmed

Withdrawal symptoms may occur during the first few days on the programme, and can sometimes last for as long as two weeks. Whilst you shouldn't definitely expect these, it's worth bearing in mind that they are very common. Depriving the body of things which it has grown used to sometimes causes it to 'bite back'. It may seem a strange concept that this should occur as a result of dietary changes. However, it is fairly similar to the mechanism of withdrawing from drugs or alcohol. Due to the possible withdrawal symptoms from certain foods and drinks, it is better not to begin this diet in your pre-menstrual phase. Make a start after your period has arrived.

Giving up tea and coffee, for example, may trigger off a number of changes in the body. These may cause you to feel tired or uptight, anxious and on edge. Headaches may occur and, more often, the desire to eat seems to persist. You will be pleased to hear that all this tends to settle down within days, certainly within a couple of weeks. Once you have passed this stage, if it happens to you at all, life becomes much easier, and before long you will notice new habit patterns forming. So much so that patients often prefer *not* to return to their former habits, simply because their tastes have changed! For example, they lose their desire for salty food and regular cups of strong coffee.

The general consensus of opinion is that it is worth persevering, for there is a light at the end of the tunnel. Our research proves this conclusively. When the Women's Nutritional Advisory Service had been in existence for one year we decided it would be desirable to get some scientific feedback on our results. We looked at the results of a group of women who had been on the programme. They had made dietary changes, taken nutritional supplements and regularly exercised. After three months 89 per cent of the women reported that they felt significantly better and there was a 91 per cent reduction in severe symptoms.

164

We are also reminded that our efforts are worthwhile by the constant flow of grateful letters we receive from patients. From reading the case histories in Part One you will have had a taste of the magnitude of the original problems and then read about incredible changes that took place. The letters we receive from women who have completed the programme often read like fairy stories. It is no wonder we are keen to see the natural approach to curing PMS being widely used!

If I haven't put you off – let's get down to it! We'll deal with dietary aspects first of all, then supplement recommendations. Just a word before we begin: it is not advisable to start following your programme during your PMS week. The reason for this is that the body can be put under strain initially when making dietary changes and it is not a good idea to have to cope with this pre-menstrually.

First of all, decide from your chart which are your main pre-menstrual symptoms. Refer to the section 'PMS and Other Related Symptoms' on page 144 and decide which vitamins and minerals you should be concentrating on in particular. Then read through the food lists starting on page 149 to familiarize yourself with the foods high in the relevant nutrient. If you are suffering severely, it's likely to encompass most of the food groups.

LET'S PUT YOU UNDER THE MICROSCOPE

Some of your symptoms fall into categories which you have now been able to identify, but for severe PMS sufferers there are often other factors which play a major part in their condition. In order to determine whether any of these factors apply to you personally, you will need to examine several groups of symptoms. I have put certain symptoms into groups to make this simpler.

On this page there is a skeleton chart for you to complete as you go along. As you read through the sections that follow, make a note of each recommendation which you feel applies to you. By the time you have finished reading the whole of Part Three of this book you should have your programme noted down for easy reference. A copy of this can be pinned up in your kitchen to remind you of the Dos and Don'ts.

PERSONAL NUTRITIONAL PROGRAMME
SUMMARY OF RECOMMENDATIONS

Diet section

1.

2.

3.

4.

5.

6.

7.

8.

9.

10.

Supplement section

1.

2.

3.

4.

5.

GENERAL RECOMMENDATIONS

There are general recommendations that should be implemented by all severe sufferers, almost regardless of which categories of PMS they suffer from. The fact that you need to cut out certain food groups now does not mean this will remain so for ever. It is simply a way of giving your body a rest and allowing it to recover. I will explain later how to go about re-introducing some of the foods into your diet.

1. Cut out caffeine

Caffeine is addictive, although we do not readily believe it to be so. It is present in tea, coffee, chocolate and cola-based drinks.

Caffeine and some other similar substances tend to aggravate PMS A symptoms, i.e. anxiety, irritability, mood swings and nervous tension. It also affects breast symptoms, and the PMS D symptoms of depression and insomnia.

It is advisable to cut caffeine out completely, and to consume only small amounts of decaffeinated coffee, as this contains other chemicals which may have an effect on PMS symptoms. Fortunately, there are many pleasant alternatives which you will find in healthfood shops.

- There are many varieties of herb tea, some fruity and some more herby in taste, most of which are caffeine-free. The most 'tea-like' substitute we have found is 'Redbush' or 'Rooibosch' tea. This can be made with or without milk. Many former tea addicts have found that after a week or two it tastes far more pleasant than ordinary tea. You will need to shop around and experiment to find teas that suit your palate.

- Dandelion coffee is certainly worth a try. It comes in instant form and in roasted root form. I like to use the root, which I put through my coffee filter.

- There are numerous other cereal alternatives you could try, all of which you should find in a good healthfood shop.

2. Reduce your dairy produce consumption

Milk, cheese, cream and yogurt tend to make PMS symptoms far worse, particularly PMS A symptoms. Keep your total daily dairy consumption down to the equivalent of one glass of milk per day. If you have a portion of cheese or a yogurt, bear in mind you have very little milk left from your allowance. There are many non-dairy sources of calcium, which you will find mentioned on the calcium food list. So there is no fear of becoming calcium-deficient.

3. Keep your salt intake to a minimum

Salt may play a part in Pre-Menstrual Syndrome. Either in the cooking or added at the table, salt leads to increased water retention which tends to aggravate many of the PMS symptoms. You should also avoid eating salty foods. A diet low in salt is a good idea for many reasons, as well as being of value in the treatment of some of your symptoms. If you have an irresistible desire for salt, try using a salt substitute high in potassium salt, rather than the commonly available sodium salt. You will find that after you have been avoiding salt for three or four weeks you no longer miss it, and will begin to taste the food itself.

4. Keep your sugar intake low

Sugar is an important dietary factor in Pre-Menstrual Syndrome. Sugar and sweet foods such as cakes, biscuits, cookies, puddings, jam (jelly), soft drinks and ice cream are high in calories (kjs) and low in important vitamins and minerals. It is deficiencies in some of these vitamins and minerals which play such a part in pre-menstrual symptoms, particularly vitamin B6 and magnesium. Having a lot of sugar in your diet may also contribute significantly to fluid retention and therefore should be avoided.

It is not widely appreciated that 'junk food' contains a lot of phosphorus, which is known to block the uptake of certain trace minerals. Without these important trace minerals PMS symptoms tend to get worse. By 'junk food' we mean processed food, refined food, prepared food, i.e. packet soups, cakes, etc. and anything that contains added sugar, such as sweets (candy), cakes, biscuits (cookies), chocolates and soft drinks.

Coming off sugar can be difficult. However, there are a number of good alternatives.

- Sweeteners can be used in drinks.

- Low-sugar or sugar-free fruit juice and nut bars can be found in many healthfood shops and used in place of sweets.

- Concentrated apple juice is a good sweetener when cooking. Small amounts of molasses may also be used as it is high in the B vitamins and magnesium.

- There are sugar-free jams (jellies) available in healthfood shops. These are made with fruit and apple juice.

- Watered-down fruit juice is a good substitute for soft drinks as it contains no extra sugar or colouring agents etc.

Unfortunately, honey consists mainly of sugar, and only one or two teaspoons should be consumed a day if you can't resist it. Similarly, small amounts of refined sugar – one teaspoon per day - may also be allowed. The same goes for brown sugar, as it has more or less the same effect on your metabolism.

There are specific supplement recommendations for sugar cravings which are mentioned on pages 183 and 188.

5. Limit your intake of alcohol

As I mentioned in Chapter 11, regular alcohol consumption can have devastating consequences on the body. Alcohol is known to block absorption of certain trace minerals and to knock out B vitamins from the system. Without these you are far more prone to pre-menstrual symptoms. Try not to consume more than two or three alcoholic drinks per week. Fortunately, there are now alcohol-free wines and beers on the market, so you need not refuse a drink.

6. Reduce cigarette smoking

Smoking may affect the levels of certain vitamins, particularly vitamin C, and also aggravate pre-menstrual breast tenderness as well as PMS A symptoms. It is advisable, therefore, that your cigarette consumption be substantially reduced. You may find it easier to cut down on smoking once you have been on the programme for a few weeks. If you don't succeed at first, try again after a month.

7. Eat your greens!

Green leafy vegetables are the major source of some important vitamins and in particular contain the mineral magnesium which plays a substantial part in the correction of pre-menstrual symptoms. It is vital, therefore, that you have a good helping of salad or green leafy vegetables every day. The greens should preferably be lightly cooked in the minimum of water to preserve their vitamin and mineral content. By careful attention to your diet, your need for vitamin and mineral supplements should be reduced.

8. Eat plenty of raw feed

Uncooked food is usually far more nutritious than food that has been cooked. In many cooking processes as much as half of the nutrients are lost. Raw food has a much higher fibre content, too. Aim to eat at least one, and preferably two raw meals per day. Eat plenty of salad stuff, fruit and raw vegetables, all of which are easy to prepare and fairly portable, if you are eating away from home. An excellent book to refer to is *Raw Energy* by Leslie and Susannah Kenton which is mentioned on the Recommended Reading List on page 252.

9. A note to vegetarians and vegans

Vegetarians who do not eat meat or fish, and vegans who only consume vegetable produce may need to pay particular attention to certain aspects of their diet, so that they do not become nutritionally deficient. Whilst there are many vegetarians who take great care over their diets, there are still too many who try to exist on lettuce leaves and the like. Apart from all the recommendations made so far, vegetarians and vegans should concentrate on the following.

Make sure you have an adequate balance of proteins in your diet.

No single vegetarian protein contains all the appropriate nutrients required, so it's important to combine the different types of vegetable proteins in your vegetarian meals. Vegetarian proteins include: nuts, seeds, peas, beans, lentils, whole grains, brown rice, sprouted beans and soya bean products.

Whilst beans are particularly nutritious, they often cause abdominal wind. Soaking them for 24 hours before cooking them and de-husking them may reduce the problem.

10. Iron and Zinc

Ensure you have an adequate intake of the minerals iron and zinc. You can check on this by referring to the iron and zinc food lists which can be found on pages 150-152.

MORE SPECIALIZED PROBLEMS: SECTIONS 1–8

I have split this section up into symptom groups. After reading through the group of symptoms, there are recommendations. If these symptoms apply to you, make a note of the recommendation on your personal chart. If the symptoms don't apply to you, then simply pass on to the next section.

Do you suffer with any of the following? (tick applicable boxes)

Abdominal bloating	☐	Depression	☐
Excessive wind	☐	Mouth ulcers	☐
Constipation	☐	Fatigue	☐
Diarrhoea	☐		

If you ticked any two of these symptoms it would be *desirable* for you to follow these recommendations.

If, however, you ticked three or more it is *advisable* for you to read through the recommendations carefully, mark them on your chart, and apply them.

SECTION 1: SENSITIVITY TO GRAINS

There is evidence to show that the symptoms mentioned in sections 1 to 8 may be related to food sensitivity. Research suggests that a significant percentage of the population produce antibodies to some foods. In our experience, this may be only a temporary state of affairs that occurs when we are not in very good nutritional shape. Finding the right kind of diet for your body will help to overcome your symptoms. It is therefore worth avoiding certain groups of foods temporarily if you suffer with the symptoms in this section. Try to follow the recommendations closely – you will reap the benefit.

WHOLEWHEAT AND GRAINS: ALTERNATIVES

Many symptoms such as irritability, abdominal bloating, constipation, diarrhoea, excessive wind, irritable bowel, fatigue and depression can be aggravated by eating foods containing wheat and other grains. Certain people react to wheat, oats, barley and rye, and all foods made from them or containing them. They are therefore better off avoiding them altogether initially, until the symptoms are under control. It sounds a bit drastic, but there are lots of alternative foods that can be used instead, so don't despair.

Bread

There are now many alternatives to ordinary bread, some of which can be purchased and others which you need to bake yourself. Both chemists and healthfood shops usually have some stocks of the alternative grain products; in our experience the chemists are usually the most reasonably priced. Behind the counter in the pharmacy you will usually find a stock of

171

products kept for people with gluten allergy. Ask the pharmacist for help, as they sometimes have to order products in on request.

Look out for some of the following products:

- Ener G white or brown rice bread (which toasts nicely)

- Glutafin wheat-free bread and rolls and Glutafin crackers

- Rice cakes

Home-made bread. Whilst I have not been very successful in making bread with alternative flours, some of our patients have successfully experimented. Look out for the recipes for potato and rice bread, and buckwheat and rice bread, on pages 210–211.

Pasta

Although you will need to avoid the pasta made with wheat, there are many reasonable alternatives you can try. Most of these are available from healthfood shops, the Chinese supermarket or the pharmacist.

- **Pastariso** make brown rice spaghetti, which is very acceptable slightly undercooked. They also do a range of other pastas. Although some healthfood shops do stock it, it is easier to order it from the chemist.

- **Glutafin** have a range of pasta which is sometimes available in healthfood shops, and again can be ordered from the chemist.

- **Rice noodles** are available in a wide variety from Chinese supermarkets. There are wide flat rice noodles that resemble tagliatelli, spaghetti-like noodles, and the very skinny variety that only need soaking in a covered pan in boiling water for a few minutes. You will probably find that these are cheaper than the alternative pastas available from healthfood shops and chemists.

Breakfast cereal

Any rice or corn cereals will be fine, even the ordinary Rice Krispies and Cornflakes from the supermarkets. Add some chopped fruit and some crumbled nuts, perhaps a few seeds and a little dried fruit to your cereal to make it a bit more wholesome. There are some alternative mueslis available, but they are usually very expensive for only a small packet.

Home-made cakes

If you enjoy cooking there are plenty of very acceptable biscuits, cakes, pastries, sponges and pancakes you can make using alternative flours. If you have never used any of the alternative flours before it may take you a little time to find the consistency that you like.

Sponge. Brown rice flour is probably the best for making sponge. Make it up to the weight given in the recipe by mixing it with a little ground almond and a raising agent (cream of tartar and bicarbonate of soda).

Raising agents. As baking powder contains wheat, you will need to use an alternative. Either use a combination of one part of bicarbonate of soda to two parts of cream of tartar, or use Glutafin wheat-free baking powder.

Savoury pancakes. These can be made with pure buckwheat flour, which is part of the rhubarb family and tends to be quite heavy, or buckwheat mixed with a little white rice flour, which is very light.

Sweet pancakes are best made with a combination of brown rice flour, or ground rice, and cornflour, purchased form a healthfood shop or Chinese supermarket. Use half cornflour and half rice flour to replace the normal quantity of flour in the ordinary pancake recipe.

Breadcrumbs or batter. A crisp coating for fish or meat can be made with maize meal, which can be found in the healthfood shop. Coat the fish or meat with maize meal, then with beaten egg, and once again with maize meal. You can then bake, grill or even fry the food which should emerge with a crispy coat.

Biscuits. There are varieties of biscuits that you can make using brown rice flour, or ground rice, and ground nuts or coconut. If you make plain biscuits you can flavour them with lemon or ginger. Our recipes for almond macaroons and coconut biscuits are very acceptable, and at the same time more nutritious than the average biscuit as they are full of eggs and nuts. It's an idea to make some and keep them in the freezer so that you can take a few out when you really feel you need something sweet to eat.

There are many other flours that you can use in your cooking. Gram flour made from chickpeas, potato flour, soya flour, tapioca flour, and millet flour are all good examples. Glutafin make flour mixes for bread, pastry and cakes, as do True Free, and these are available in some health-food shops.

Shop-bought cakes and biscuits

Acceptable cakes and biscuits can now be purchased in healthfood shops and ordered from most chemists.

Glutafin have a range of biscuits including digestives, and Rite-Diet have a range of biscuits and cakes. The coconut biscuits are the least sweet, and the banana or lemon cakes are worth trying too.

Snacks

It's nice to have something to crunch on when you are avoiding wheat. There are lots of corn products available, but do remember to read the labels as some have added wheat. Try corn chips, crisps, and wafers, and look in the Mexican section of the supermarket. Also, poppadoms are fine, and little mini spiced poppadoms are nice to nibble on or dip.

ASSESSING FOR GRAIN SENSITIVITY

You will need to become a nutritional detective by doing the following:

- Stop eating all the grains mentioned earlier (wheat, oats, barley, rye) for at least a month, preferably six weeks. You can eat one slice of French bread per day if you are desperate! But it's better to try to manage on rice crackers or rice cakes instead. This may seem strange as refined bread is nowhere near as nutritious as wholemeal bread. However, during the refining process most of the grain has been removed and therefore the degree of aggravation caused by this is far less than by a wholegrain loaf.

- After a month or six weeks, or longer, when you feel that your symptoms have diminished, try introducing the various grains one by one to your diet. Begin just after a period, so that you don't confuse any reaction with PMS symptoms. Choose one grain, e.g. rye in the form of Ryvita. Introduce this into your diet and eat this for several days. If you have no reaction after five days, choose another grain and repeat this process. *DO NOT MIX the grains initially* because if you do get a reaction you won't know exactly what you have reacted to! Continue to do this with all the grains, providing you don't have reactions to any one of them. Try wheat last as it is the most common grain to cause problems.

Once you get used to using the alternatives you shouldn't find the diet difficult to stick to. If you are going to avoid eating certain groups of foods for any length of time, it is important to arm yourself with all the alternative foods you can muster. It is not a weight-loss diet (although you might find that you lose weight if you are overweight) and you can literally eat as much as you like of the foods on your list. Never allow yourself to get hungry and never miss a meal. It's important to keep up a steady flow of good nutrients in order to allow your hormone and brain chemical metabolism to function at an optimum.

What to do if you have a reaction

The reactions may include diarrhoea or constipation, excessive wind, abdominal bloating, headaches, weight gain, fatigue, confusion, depression, mouth ulcers, rash, irritability and palpitations.

1. Once you have established what you have reacted to, make a note of it and avoid eating this food at all for now. This doesn't mean that you won't be able to eat this food again ever, but it is best avoided for now.

2. Wait until things have settled down again and then try again with another grain.

I appreciate that cutting out all grains is a severe measure. I suggest you begin by just cutting out wholewheat products. You will need to do this for at least four to six weeks to see whether there is any improvement. You can remain on small amounts of white or French bread.

Constipation

If constipation is a particular problem you might like to try taking some linseed. You can find some very palatable forms of it at your healthfood shop such as Linusit Gold. It is pleasant to eat and can easily be included in your breakfast cereals or salad.

Foods containing grains

It's surprising how many foods contain grains. Before I began 'label reading' I would never have believed the extent to which grains are used. It's a good exercise to go around the supermarket, reading labels on packets to get an idea of this for yourself. Sometimes labels aren't as explicit as they might be and they just contain the words 'edible starch'. This has to be regarded with suspicion if you are on a grain-free diet. Labelling of food in healthfood shops is usually more reliable and precise.

Wheat. The most obvious foods containing wheat are bread, biscuits, cakes and flour made from wheat etc., but wheat is often present in pre-pared sauces, soups, and processed foods in general. Gluten-free products are not particularly recommended on a wheat-free diet as some of them still contain wheat.

The following list will give you a rough idea of what to look out for, but I suggest you make a practice of reading labels thoroughly before buying anything.

- Bread, particularly wholemeal, wheatmeal, etc. as these contain more of the natural wheat.

- Cakes, biscuits, pasta, spaghetti, macaroni etc. – pastry, pies, buns, bran (except rice or soya bran), and many breakfast cereals and sausages.

Oats. Porridge, oat cookies and oat flakes.

Rye. Rye bread (which may also contain wheat), Ryvita.

Barley. Often found in packet/tinned soups and stews, barley beverages.

Corn. Corn on the cob, corn starch, corn (maize), oil and popcorn.

There are many lovely recipe books available with further ideas listed in the Recommended Reading section on page 251.

I have prepared some sample menus to give you an idea of the scope pos-sible. There are also a few recipes included in the recipe section on page 193 as a guideline.

GRAIN FREE ALLERGY DIET

SAMPLE DAILY MENU – WHEAT, OATS, BARLEY AND RYE FREE

Breakfast

Cornflakes or Rice Krispies with:
    a piece of chopped fruit (e.g. a banana, some grapes, berries etc.)
    a few crumbled pecan nuts
    a tablespoon of pine nuts
    a tablespoon of raisins (if not avoiding yeast)
with milk *or* yogurt

Followed by:

One or two slices of alternative toast with low sugar jam or marmalade

Alternatively:

2 scrambled eggs *or* omelette with grilled tomatoes
or boiled or poached eggs
Alternative crackers and low sugar spreads

Mid-morning snack
See **Snack list** overleaf.

Lunch
Jacket potato with a nutritious filling, for example:
    Tuna and sweetcorn with a little sour cream and black pepper
    Prawns
    Baked beans
    Curried chicken

or

Cold meat *or* fresh or tinned fish with salad

or

Rice noodles, *or* alternative pasta, and vegetables

or

Home-made soup and salad

Tea-time snack
See **Snack list** overleaf.

Dinner
Poultry/fish/meat or vegetarian protein served with three portions of vegetables.

Fresh fruit or a fresh fruit salad, or choose an appropriate sweet from the dessert section in this book starting on page 208 or from the *Beat PMT Cookbook*.

Snack list

raw vegetables and dips like humus, taramasalata or guacamole
fresh fruit, nuts or seeds
yogurt and fruit
alternative crackers and spreads
corn chips
mini poppadoms
rice salad with fruit and nuts

Beverages

Coffee substitutes. Dandelion coffee, chicory, or up to two cups of decaffeinated coffee per day.

Herbal teas. Rooibosch Eleven O'clock tea (with milk). This herbal tea 'look alike', available from healthfood shops, contains a mild, natural muscle relaxant and may help alleviate tension and ease period pains. It is favoured by many of our patients and is definitely worth a try. Other suggestions are bramble, raspberry and ginseng, mixed berry, lemon verbena, fennel and wild strawberry. These days most healthfood shops sell single sachets so that you can 'buy and try' without being saddled with a whole box of tea bags that you absolutely detest.

Cold drinks. Bottled water with or without fruit juice, mineral water, Appletise, Rio, or Citrus Spring.

B = Breakfast   L = Lunch   D = Dinner   S = Sweet

For recipes, see Chapter 17, page 193.

A SAMPLE MENU PLAN FOR ONE WEEK

DAY 1

B   Orange juice
     Buckwheat pancakes (crêpes)
     Dried fruit conserve
L   Fresh avocado and tomato
       soup
     Jacket potato with cheese
D   Cold mackerel fillets or
       Prince's Mackerel in Spicy
       Tomato Sauce
     Green salad

     Brown rice salad
S   Baked stuffed apples

DAY 2

B   ½ grapefruit
     Mushroom omelette
L   Sliced turkey
     Orange and beanshoot salad
     Banana

D   Stir-fry vegetables and brown
    rice
S   Grain-free carrot cake

DAY 3
B   Apple juice
    Orange and apple salad with
    millet flakes and nuts
L   Stuffed tomatoes
    Waldorf salad (using
    sunflower seeds and nuts)
D   Grilled trout
    Green leafy vegetables
    Carrots and parsnips in herb
    sauce (thickened with
    potato flour)
    Boiled potatoes
S   Banana cream

DAY 4
B   ½ grapefruit
    Hot fruit breakfast
L   Tuna omelette
    Salad
D   Rosemary and garlic lamb
    Brown rice
    Jacket potato garnished with
    (bell) peppers and parsley
S   Slice of apple cake

DAY 5
B   Orange juice
    Buckwheat pancakes (crêpes)

    with tomatoes, (bell)
    pepper and herbs
L   Leek soup
    Jacket potato with prawns
    (shrimps)
    Plums
D   Roast chicken
    Leaf greens
    Carrots
    Sprouts and turnips
    Boiled potatoes
S   Dried fruit compote and
    yogurt

DAY 6
B   ½ grapefruit
    Smoked haddock
    Mushrooms, tomatoes
L   Green salad
    Rice salad and dressing
    Apple
D   Liver and onions
    Green vegetables
    Sauté potatoes
S   Fruity cakes

DAY 7
B   Cornflakes
    Banana, sliced
    Crumbled pecan nuts
    1 tbsp raisins
    Yogurt or milk
L   Savoury buckwheat pancakes
    (crêpes) with salmon, tuna
    or mackerel filling
D   Colourful lentils and salad
S   Fruit jelly

Snacks

With attention focused very much on food, you may get the 'munchies' for a few weeks. There are a number of things to eat between meals which will prevent you from dipping into the cookie jar!

1. Rice crackers or rice cakes from the healthfood shop. The crackers are particularly nice spread with peanut butter, sesame spread or sugar-free jam (jelly), all these from healthfood shops, too.

2. Sesame seeds or other seeds from healthfood shops are pleasant to nibble between meals.

3. Unsalted nuts can be eaten freely, but limit intake of peanuts, which are somewhat indigestible.

4. Fruit of your choice.

5. Rice biscuits or sesame biscuits and healthfood bars that don't contain wheat. Watch out for the sugar, though!

SECTION 2: SENSITIVITY TO YEAST

Do you suffer from any of the following symptoms?

Thrush (more than two episodes in the last five years) ☐	Cracking at the corners of your mouth ☐
	Depression ☐
Itchy bottom ☐	Excessive wind ☐
Bloated abdomen ☐	Cystitis ☐

Two or more episodes of thrush and/or any other two symptoms certainly qualify you for the yeast-free diet.

YEAST SENSITIVITY

Yeast problems in the gut are very common it seems, and they can produce or aggravate a wide variety of symptoms. Everyone has the yeast bug in their gut in harmless quantities (*candida albicans*), but in many people it gets triggered into rapid growth, producing toxins which then affect us, often without our realizing.

180

A few of the symptoms are of the emotional, mental and physical variety. These are also often 'allergic' type symptoms.

The more obvious yeast conditions are thrush in the vagina or in the mouth, cystitis, abdominal bloating and flatulence.

Many PMS symptoms seem to be aggravated by the yeast bug, *candida*. The vague symptoms of confusion, fatigue, lethargy, depression, poor memory, the feeling of 'not really being there' etc. – the list seems endless.

There are several actions that can be taken to prevent this problem continuing.

Avoiding yeast in food

It is surprising how many foods contain yeast. Yeast is used frequently in food preparation processes, in which case it is generally marked on the label of the product. However, yeast is a fungus which grows on food, particularly left-over food, even if well covered. It is also particularly fond of foods with an acid-base like citrus fruits and vinegar.

The following list is a guide to foods high in yeast, which you should try to avoid if you want to reduce the PMS symptoms mentioned above.

1. All foods containing sugar or honey, as yeast thrives on sugary or starchy food.

2. All bread, buns, biscuits, cakes etc.

3. Most alcoholic drinks often depend on yeasts to produce the alcohol, especially beer.

4. Citrus fruit juices – only fresh home-squeezed juice is yeast-free.

5. Malted cereals, malted drinks.

6. Pickles, sauerkraut, olives, chilli peppers.

7. Blue cheese (Roquefort).

8. Mushrooms and mushroom sauce.

9. Hamburgers, sausages and cooked meats made with bread or breadcrumbs. Yeast extract (Miso).

10. All fermented foods.

11. Dried fruits.

12. Left-over or stale food.

13. Vitamins. All B-vitamin preparations are likely to be derived from

yeast unless otherwise stated; but most manufacturers do make some B-vitamin preparations which are free of yeasts.

Other contributory factors

Apart from dietary changes there are a few other areas to check. The Pill can make yeast problems worse and should be avoided. Advice should be sought from the Family Planning Clinic for an alternative method of contraception. If the symptoms persist you may need to consult your doctor.

Hints for beating thrush

- Wear cotton underwear instead of nylon.

- Douche with live yogurt for immediate relief.

- Get your sexual partner treated as well, as it is highly likely that you would pass it back and forwards to each other.

There are some very helpful books on the subject of yeast problems on page 251.

ANITA'S THRUSH PROBLEMS

'I had continual thrush. I had been under my doctor for this problem and we had tried everything but nothing handled it. I had oral tablets, pessaries to insert in the vagina, creams etc. I tried using live yogurt and even baby oil; I changed my underwear and even stopped wearing tights. Nothing made an impression on the thrush until it was suggested that my diet was continually aggravating the thrush and I went on the nutritional programme. I was asked to stick to the recommendations strictly and my thrush cleared up completely. Wheat does make a difference to me. I'm okay now if I have one or two slices of bread or a small amount of cereal, but if I go beyond that I'll start to bloat. The minute I had a little alcohol as well back would come my thrush. So when I get the feeling I'm going to develop it, I cut out all foods containing yeast. I used to be absolutely plagued with thrush. It has totally vanished now, I haven't had any reoccurrence for at least 18 months.'

GERALDINE'S THRUSH PROBLEMS

'I had thrush all the time before I went on the programme. The hospital gave me a prescription and told me to use it for three months and not to have any sexual contact with my husband whatsoever in the meantime! Our marriage was already going through a very rough phase at this point, and I'd already tried this treatment before. I tried using the treatment again. It helped for a bit, but as soon as I stopped it the thrush was worse than ever. I had more pessaries and even went into hospital where it was suggested I paint the affected area violet. Diet certainly did help. Once I cut out sugary foods and other yeast-based foods it made a tremendous difference and the thrush began to clear up by itself.'

SECTION 3: HEADACHES

Do you suffer from the following?

Migraine headaches? ☐

Regular pre-menstrual headaches? ☐

Migraine symptoms may be aggravated by cheese, alcohol, oranges, tea, coffee, chocolate, fermented foods, potted foods and pastes, yeast and wholemeal (wholewheat) bread, smoked and preserved food and yeast extract. It is therefore advisable to avoid these foods where possible for at least a period of two to three months to see whether it makes any difference to your symptoms.

Make sure any vitamin supplements you take are yeast-free.

SECTION 4: SUGAR CRAVINGS

Do you suffer with excessive sugar cravings? There are several things you can do if sugar cravings are a problem.

- Sugar cravings could well improve by taking particular supplements, including vitamin B complex, magnesium and the mineral chromium. Chromium deals with sugar balance in the body, and thus plays an important and effective role in controlling sugar cravings.

- Eat a diet rich in foods containing chromium (see page 154).

183

- Whilst you are experiencing the sugar cravings, eat little and often. In other words, have five or six smaller meals per day, rather than three larger ones. This will help your blood sugar to remain constant and prevent you from having the extreme sugar cravings.

SECTION 5: IRON DEFICIENCY

Do you suffer with the following?

Heavy periods	☐	Cracking at the corners of the mouth	☐
Fatigue	☐	A sore tongue	☐

Heavy periods alone can cause iron deficiency. The other symptoms mentioned above may serve to confirm this. IUDs can sometimes cause heavy bleeding, so if you have a coil, it might be advisable to have a check-up and possibly consider an alternative method of contraception.

With any of the above symptoms you would be wise to ask your doctor to check your serum iron, to see whether you may need some iron supplements. In the meantime you should concentrate on eating iron-rich foods (see page 151).

SECTION 6: ZINC DEFICIENCY

Do you suffer with any of the following?

Acne	☐	Eczema	☐
White spots on your nails	☐	Poor hair growth	☐
Split brittle nails	☐	Infertility	☐

Any combination of the above symptoms may indicate that you need to increase your intake of zinc. This can be done by concentrating on foods rich in zinc and initially by taking a zinc supplement.

184

SECTION 7: FATTY ACID DEFICIENCY

Do you have any of the following?

Dry rough pimply skin on the upper arms or thighs ☐	Dandruff	☐
Red greasy skin ☐	Dry flaky skin	☐
	Eczema	☐

These symptoms may indicate that you are short of essential fatty acids. If you feel this may be so, you can refer to the Food List on essential fats on page 155. Evening primrose oil capsules may be helpful, as is cold pressed linseed oil when taken orally.

SECTION 8: BREAST TENDERNESS

Do you suffer with severe breast tenderness or lumpy breasts pre-menstrually? There are a number of preventive measures you can take:

- Eat a low salt diet.

- Cut out tea and coffee.

- Cut out cigarettes, or at least cut down.

- Restrict your dairy produce intake.

- Keep alcohol consumption to a minimum.

- If taking the contraceptive pill it might be worth changing your Pill or using an alternative method of contraception.

TAKE ONE STEP AT A TIME

There are many new ideas for you to absorb. If you don't feel you can make the necessary changes all at once, then make them gradually. The closer you follow the recommendations, the better off you are likely to feel after you have overcome any withdrawal symptoms that may occur at the very beginning.

It's quite normal to feel sceptical about the value of making such drastic changes. It is only when you start to feel better that you are likely to believe that this is a workable solution.

WILL YOU BE ON A RESTRICTED DIET FOR EVER?

There seems to be a definite difference between a 'food allergy' and a 'food sensitivity'. More often than not we find that severe PMS cases are suffering with food sensitivity rather than actual allergy, although there are cases where women are violently allergic to certain types of food.

Realistically, if you are suffering with severe symptoms, you need to give your body a complete rest for a minimum of two to three months. We often find it takes as much as six months to a year before the body is really back to normal, and can once again cope fully with foods that have been eliminated.

If you notice unpleasant side-effects occurring when you begin to reintroduce the grains, one by one, or products containing yeast, discontinue them for another month or two, before attempting to reintroduce them again. Usually, the very fact that there is so much progress occurring is an incentive to continue with the nutritional programme.

Occasionally we have found that some unfortunate souls have what seems to be a permanent allergy to a particular food, which when reintroduced continues to make them feel very unwell. In these cases the women themselves usually decide that it is better to be well and do without the food in question than to suffer unnecessarily.

It is probably better not to reintroduce foods to your diet during your pre-menstrual week. I usually suggest waiting until your period is over and you are feeling at your best.

CHEATING

One for one, the women who go through the programme cheat at some point. Not only do we expect it, we also think it is a positive step. It's only when you have put the system to the test yourself that you really begin to follow it because you believe in it, rather than following it because someone else said it might work.

I have to smile when I think of the stories I'm told about broken diets. I've been through restricted diets myself, so I know what happens. It goes like this. You begin to feel so well on the diet, in fact you've almost forgotten how rotten you felt initially. Amazing how the memory of pain and discomfort evaporates!

You begin to doubt that you really have food sensitivities, perhaps it's just a coincidence that you felt 'unwell' at the time you were eating your favourite restricted food. So you decide to blow the diet. You eat and enjoy one or two days' helpings of the forbidden 'fruit'. Sometimes the symptoms return within an hour or two, sometimes they creep on within a day or so; either way, you have the symptoms back again and you remember what feeling so unwell was like. You now realize that dietary factors and your symptoms are clearly related. So it's back on the diet with a far more self-determined resolution not to cheat!

IN THE LONG TERM

Once you have been following the dietary and supplement recommendations closely for three or four months, and you have noticed substantial improvement, you can then start to relax a bit. As long as you follow the basic recommendations most of the time, the occasional indulgence shouldn't hurt. Make sure it's only occasional to begin with, and preferably not in the pre-menstrual week. As a general rule, supplements should not be necessary in the long term. They should be taken until you feel that your symptoms are well under control. This may take as little as three or four months or as long as nine months to a year.

Occasionally, months after completing your programme, symptoms may recur. Times of great stress and general illness may, in some circumstances place extra nutritional demands on your body and this may bring on some of the old symptoms. Should this happen to you, identify which PMS category they fall into and take the appropriate dietary action. Use your original programme to help you.

Again, as symptoms reduce, gradually return to the maintenance recommendations and reduce the supplements gradually. It is important to do this in stages as abrupt withdrawal can often lead to recurrence of symptoms.

Do remember to take action quickly with any symptoms so that they can be relieved quickly.

STEP 3 – CHOOSING YOUR SUPPLEMENTS

We never advise women to take random supplements without some sort of advice. Our bodies are fairly sensitive mechanisms which have specific needs. Too much of a particular nutrient can cause imbalances and consequently other problems in the long term.

Before considering supplements, have a look at the chart called 'Physical Signs of Vitamin and Mineral Deficiency' on page 189: you might recognize some of the signs of vitamin and mineral deficiency which you have had for years but accepted as being 'normal'.

PHYSICAL SIGNS OF
VITAMIN AND MINERAL DEFICIENCIES

There are several useful supplements that can be tried in conjunction with each other. Assuming your symptoms are fairly severe and you are looking for the most effective treatment I will first sugest the optimum regime to begin on, regardless of cost. I will then go on to discuss cheaper, and finally, still cheaper alternatives. As you decide which supplements to try, make a note of their name and the daily dosage on your personal tailor-made programme.

MULTI-VITAMIN AND MINERAL SUPPLEMENTS

The first and most basic supplement to take is a multi-vitamin and mineral supplement which contains goodly amounts of the essential nutrients mentioned.

The most tried and tested multi-vitamin and mineral supplement for PMS is an American supplement, formulated by Dr Guy Abraham, Optivite for Women. It has been through several American clinical trials and has been shown to raise progesterone levels. It is available in the USA and the UK.

The Women's Nutritional Advisory Service has conducted two trials on Optivite, the results of which are detailed on page 191.

We usually recommend that four tablets be taken per day during the first few months. After this, reduce down to two per day until mid cycle, increasing to four per day during your pre-menstrual time. Sometimes, in severe cases, six tablets should be taken per day. If your symptoms are moderate, then a lower dosage may be used.

Another multi-vitamin and mineral supplement that performed well in a clinical trial is Femvite. This new supplement is based on WNAS research and is considerably cheaper than Optivite. It is currently available from Nutritional Health (mail order) and is expected to be available from chemists and healthfood shops by late 1994.

There are certain situations when other supplements need to be taken alongside your multi-vitamin and mineral tablets, some of these are listed on the chart on page 190.

PHYSICAL SIGNS OF
VITAMIN AND MINERAL DEFICIENCY

Sign or Symptom	Can be Caused by Deficiencies of:
Cracking at the corners of the mouth	Iron, vitamins B12, B6, Folic acid
Recurrent mouth ulcers	Iron, vitamins B12, B6, Folic acid
Dry, cracked lips	Vitamin B2
Smooth (sore) tongue	Iron, vitamins B2, B12, Folic acid
Enlargement/prominence of taste buds at tip of the tongue (red, sore)	Vitamins B2, or B6
Red, greasy skin on face, especially sides of nose	Vitamins B2, B6, zinc or essential fatty acids
Rough, sometimes red, pimply skin on upper arms and thighs	Vitamin B complex, vitamin E or essential fatty acids
Skin conditions such as eczema, dry, rough, cracked, peeling skin	Zinc, essential fatty acids
Poor hair growth	Iron or zinc
Dandruff	Vitamin C, vitamin B6, zinc, essential fatty acids
Acne	Zinc
Bloodshot, gritty, sensitive eyes	Vitamins A or B2
Night blindness	Vitamin A or zinc
Dry eyes	Vitamin A, essential fatty acids
Brittle or split nails	Iron, zinc or essential fatty acids
White spots on nails	Zinc
Pale appearance due to anaemia	Iron, vitamin B12, Folic acid, essential to consult your doctor

Problem	Type of Supplement	Daily Dosage	Available from
*PMS, A, H, C, D	Optivite or Femvite	2–6 tabs daily	Boots, chemists, healthfood shops and Nutritional Health (mail order)
*Breast problems	Efamol/Efamast evening primrose oil Natural Vitamin E	4-8 500 mg capsules daily 400 IUs daily	Chemists, healthfood shops, Nutritional Health (mail order) and prescription
Extreme nervous tension, drug withdrawals	Strong Vitamin B complex	1–2 tabs daily	Healthfood shops
*Sugar cravings	Normoglycaemia/ Sugar Factor	1–2 tabs daily	Nutritional Health (mail order)
*Eczema	Efamol/Epogam evening primrose oil	4–8 500 mg tabs daily	Boots, chemists, healthfood shops, Nutritional Health (mail order) and prescription
Dry, rough skin/ dandruff	Cold pressed linseed oil	2 tbsp with fruit juice at night	Healthfood shops
*Period pains/ palpitations insomnia	Magnesium chelate or magnesium hydroxide mixture	2 500 mg tabs daily or 15 ml taken as 5 ml 3 times daily	Healthfood shops and chemists

*Available by mail order through Nutritional Health,
 PO Box 926 Lewes, East Sussex BN7 2QL.

IMPORTANT POINTS

- Never take supplements without the consent of your GP if you have a current medical problem.

- Always begin taking your supplements gradually. For example, if you are due to take two or four per day of a particular supplement, begin taking them one tablet per day and gradually build up to the optimum dosage over the period of a week or two. Take them after meals unless otherwise specified.

How to cut down on your supplements

- Cut down on the dosage very gradually over a period of months rather than weeks, but keep taking the supplements each day of your cycle.

- Once you have reduced the dosage gradually, if you feel that your symptoms are well under control you can leave the supplements off altogether the week after your period.

190

- After another couple of months you can remain supplement-free for two weeks after your period.

- You might prefer to keep taking supplements pre-menstrually, or to cut them out completely and only take them at times of great stress. Some women prefer to take small doses daily on a permanent basis. There is no harm in doing so. As you will probably recognize from Chapter 11, which deals with our diet today, the nutrients in our food are often lost to us, therefore taking supplements in the long term as a general health aid may be a sensible move.

RESULTS OF CLINICAL TRIALS PERFORMED BY THE PRE-MENSTRUAL TENSION ADVISORY SERVICE

Name and type of product	Available from	Dosage given	Improved a lot	Improved slightly	No worse but no better
Optivite	Nature's Best	4 per day increasing to 8 per day pre-menstrually	71.5%	16.5%	12%
Optivite	Nature's Best	2 per day increasing to 4 pre-menstrually	65%	31%	6%
Evening primrose oil (Efamol)	Healthfood shops	8×500 mg capsules per day	64%	19%	17%
Femvite	Chemists, mail order (available from health-food shops in late 1994)	2 per day	84%	7%	7%
PMT	Australia New Zealand Singapore	2 per day	60%	30%	10%

Out of all the supplements available, only Optivite and Efamol have shown consistently significant results in clinical trials. For details of supplements available in Australia and New Zealand see Appendix 3.

WHAT ABOUT YOUR DRUGS?

If you are currently taking prescribed drugs from your doctor, I don't advise you to stop taking them or reduce them without his or her consent. Having said that, we do find that most women, once established on their nutritional programme, no longer feel the need for their tranquillizers, anti-depressants or sleeping pills.

Vitamins and minerals can be taken quite happily alongside most drugs. There are a few exceptions however. Any antibiotic in the tetracycline family should not be taken with minerals. Evening primrose oil should not be taken by anyone who has a history of epilepsy. When you feel the time has come to reduce your drugs, do go to see your doctor before taking any action, especially if you have been taking the drugs for a long period of time. Coming off drugs suddenly may bring on nasty withdrawal symptoms.

17

NUTRITIOUS RECIPES

Although this is not designed to be a recipe book, I felt it would be useful for you to have some guidelines to work with. It's better if you are not short of ideas to begin with: the more you like your new diet, the higher the chances of your sticking to it. In the Recommended Reading List on page 251, I have suggested many inexpensive recipe books which will give you further ideas. It might be an idea to visit a good bookshop and have a browse through the books, so that you can select those you find most suitable.

The recipes I have given cover breakfast, soups, lunch, dinner and sweets. All the recipes are suitable for those of you who are moderate sufferers. For those of you who suffer severely and therefore select a restricted diet, follow the recipes with a code beside them.

There are two codes:

G = Grain-free.
Y = Low yeast content.
No code = Suitable for all sufferers who are not on restricted diets.

Note: Imperial and American measures are given in brackets, where appropriate.
  Use salt substitute, not salt.
  Miso when not in brackets is soya.

BREAKFASTS

WHOLEWHEAT PANCAKES (CREPES)

110 g (4 oz/½ cup) wholemeal (wholewheat or buckwheat) flour
1 small egg

300 ml (10 fl oz/1¼ cups) skimmed (skim) milk
oil for cooking

Make a thin batter with the flour, egg and skimmed milk, whisking well. Use kitchen paper to wipe a small non-stick frying pan with oil and heat until it is smoking. Pour a generous 2 tablespoons of the batter into the pan and swirl it around to cover bottom as thinly as possible. Cook the batter for 60 seconds, then flip it over with a spatula and cook the other side for a few seconds only. If you are going to eat straight away, tip on to a heated plate – otherwise, stacked pancakes with cling film (plastic wrap) in between can be stored in the refrigerator. They can be easily reheated individually on a plate covered with foil over a pan of water, or in the microwave oven. SERVES 4

MUESLI

½ mug (½ cup) dried apricots
½ mug (½ cup) jumbo oats
½ mug (½ cup) barley flakes
¼ mug (¼ cup) large sultanas
   (golden raisins)

½ pint (1 cup) fresh orange juice
2 apples, grated
milk to mix
¼ mug (¼ cup) chopped mixed nuts
clear honey, to taste

Put apricots, oats, barley flakes, sultanas and orange juice in a mixing bowl. Cover and leave to soak overnight. Next morning, stir in the apple and sufficient milk to give a soft consistency. Spoon the muesli into dishes and top with chopped nuts and honey. SERVES 3–4

HOT FRUITY BREAKFAST

25 g (1 oz/2 tbsp) lightly crushed millet, toasted

150 ml (¼ pint/½ cup) milk
stewed fruit according to taste

Mix the millet and milk in a pan. Bring gently to the boil and simmer for 5 minutes, stirring occasionally. Put in a serving bowl, stir in 15–30 ml (1–2 tbsp) stewed fruit, and serve with extra milk substitute or a spoonful of sugar-free jam. SERVES 1

DRIED FRUIT CONSERVE G

200 g (7 oz/1 cup) dried apricots	or
apple juice	5 ml (1 tsp) grated orange peel
Use one of the following	or
flavourings:	50 g (2 oz/½ cup) flaked almonds
5 ml (1 tsp) orange flower water	

Soak apricots overnight in water. Put the apricots into a saucepan and just cover them with apple juice, using the minimum amount to ensure a thick purée. Simmer them, uncovered, for about 30 minutes or until they are thoroughly cooked and soft. Cool and then thoroughly blend or sieve them until they have a smooth, thick consistency. Add one of the flavourings.

Purée will keep in refrigerator for about 10 days. SERVES 2

SOUPS

LENTIL AND VEGETABLE SOUP   G

15 g (½ oz) soft vegetable margarine	100 g (4 oz) cabbage, shredded
1 onion, chopped	100 g (4 oz/½ cup) continental
1 garlic clove, crushed	lentils, pre-soaked
2 large carrots, finely diced	1 litre (1¾ pints) vegetable stock
2 sticks celery, sliced	bouquet garni (sprig parsley, thyme
2 tomatoes, skinned and chopped	and bay leaf tied)
50 g (2 oz/1 cup) mushrooms,	parsley
chopped	pepper

Melt margarine in a large saucepan and sauté the onion for five minutes without browning. Add garlic and rest of vegetables and cook gently for five minutes over the heat, then add the stock and bouquet garni, stir in extra parsley and season to taste with pepper. SERVES 4

195

BROCCOLI SOUP   G&Y

225 g (8 oz–1 lb) broccoli, chopped
1.7 litres (3 pints) vegetable stock
1.25 ml (¼ tsp) salt

30 ml (2 tbsp) semi-skimmed (skim)
  milk
pinch nutmeg
pinch cayenne pepper

Combine broccoli, stock and salt in large saucepan, bring to the boil. Reduce heat and simmer for 15 minutes. Remove from heat, blend mixture to purée with milk, nutmeg and cayenne. Return to pan, heat through, do not boil. SERVES 6

NUTTY PARSNIP SOUP   G

25 g (1 oz/1 tbsp) vegetable
  margarine
1 medium onion, chopped
300 g (10½ oz) parsnips, sliced
1 tbsp smooth peanut butter

dash shoyu (soya derivative, from
  healthfood shops)
1 vegetable stock cube
600 ml (1 pint) water
25 g (1 oz/¼ cup) peanuts, roasted

Melt the margarine in a deep pan. Sauté the onions and parsnips together until beginning to soften. Stir in the peanut butter to coat the vegetables. Add a little shoyu. Bring vegetable stock to the boil and add the water gradually, allowing the peanut butter to thicken slightly. Continue cooking until all ingredients are soft. Blend. Roughly grate the peanuts and scatter on the surface just before serving. (Hazelnuts and hazelnut butter can be used instead.) SERVES 4

FRESH AVOCADO AND TOMATO SOUP   G&Y

50 g (2 oz/¼ stick) butter/margarine
1 medium-sized onion, chopped
1 small potato, chopped
450 g (1 lb) tomatoes, quartered
2 garlic cloves

1 bay leaf
30 ml (2 tbsp) tomato purée (paste)
450 ml (¾ pint) vegetable stock
450 ml (¾ pint) milk
2 avocados (ripe)
pepper to taste

Melt the butter/margarine and sauté the onion until transparent. Add potato, tomatoes, garlic, bay leaf, tomato paste and stock. Cover and simmer for 20 minutes. Take off the heat, stirring in the milk and chopped avocado flesh. Remove bay leaf. Blend in small quantities in liquidizer goblet. Adjust seasoning to taste and reheat to serving temperature. SERVES 4–6

CHICKEN SOUP   G&Y

1 chicken boned and cut into 2.5 cm (1 in) cubes

600 ml (1 pint) water

4 garlic cloves, sliced (optional, to taste)

2 sticks of celery, chopped

2 carrots, chopped

1 medium onion

50 g (2 oz) peas

50 g (2 oz) cooked brown rice

25 g (1 oz) parsley, chopped

herbs and seasoning to taste

Simmer chicken in water for 40 minutes. Add garlic, vegetables and rice and simmer for additional 20 minutes. Serve topped with scissor-snipped fresh parsley. Add herbs according to taste. SERVES 4

SALADS

Always use the very best and freshest ingredients.

BEANSHOOT SALAD   G&Y

50 g (2 oz/½ cup) almond halves

1 tsp oil

¼ tsp salt

50 g (2 oz) carrots

2 bananas

300 g (8 oz) fresh beanshoots

Put the almonds, oil and salt in small ovenproof dish. Mix well, then roast in the oven at 200°C (400°F/Mark 6) for about 10 minutes until golden. Leave until cold. Grate carrots and slice the bananas, combine with almonds and beanshoots. SERVES 4

WALDORF SALAD   G

4 sticks celery

50 g (2 oz/½ cup) walnuts

1 large dessert apple

150 g (6 oz) Cheddar cheese

salt and pepper

French dressing

Chop the celery and walnuts. Dice the apple and cheese. Mix all the ingredients together in a salad bowl. Add seasoning and dressing to taste. SERVES 4

BULGAR AND NUT SALAD

200 g (8 oz/1⅓ cups) bulgar
 (cracked wheat)
1 large sized onion, finely chopped
3 tbsp olive oil
100 ml (4 fl oz) tomato purée
 (paste)
60 ml (4 tbsp) dried mint

5 ml (1 tsp) ground cumin
5 ml (1 tsp) ground coriander
2.5 ml (½ tsp) ground allspice
110 g (4 oz/1 cup) walnuts and/or
 hazelnuts, very coarsely chopped
juice of 1 lemon

Soak the cracked wheat (available from healthfood shops) in plenty of fresh cold water for 15 minutes, drain it well and squeeze out as much of the water as you can. Fry the chopped onion in a tablespoon of oil, until very soft but not yet coloured. Mix all the ingredients in a large serving bowl and leave for about an hour for the bulgar to absorb the flavours and become plump and tender. SERVES 4

GRAPEFRUIT AND ORANGE SALAD   G&Y

1 whole grapefruit
1 orange
75 g (3 oz/½ cup) sunflower seeds

50 g (2 oz/½ cup) mixed nuts
 chopped
orange juice, freshly squeezed

Remove rind of grapefruit and orange and chop flesh, mix with sunflower seeds and nuts and a little orange juice. SERVES 4

ORANGE AND CUCUMBER SALAD   G&Y

2 oranges, divided into segments
½ cucumber, thinly sliced

1 small onion, thinly sliced into rings
½ small lettuce

Mix all ingredients together. SERVES 4

GREEN BEAN AND SWEETCORN SALAD   Y

200 g (8 oz) young French beans,
   topped and tailed
150 g (6 oz) can sweetcorn

2 spring onions (scallions), thinly
   sliced
2 tbsp French dressing (not for low
   yeast diet)

Cook the beans in slightly salted boiling water until tender. Drain, refresh
in cold running water, leave to cool. Mix together the beans, sweetcorn
and onions, Stir together with French dressing. SERVES 4

SALAD DRESSINGS

PEANUT AND CHILLI   G

25 ml (1 fl oz/2 tbsp) peanut oil
1 medium onion, thinly sliced
2.5 ml (½ tsp) chilli powder
5 ml (1 tsp) sugar/honey
5 ml (1 tsp) shoyu/tamari (soy
   sauce, from healthfood shops)
15 ml (1 tbsp) tomato purée (paste)
   (optional)

30–45 ml (2–3 tbsp) peanut butter
   (smooth)
3 cloves garlic, crushed or finely
   chopped
200 ml (7 fl oz/1 cup) water
200 ml (7 fl oz/1 cup) milk
dash of pepper

Heat oil gently and stir in onion, chilli, sugar/honey and shoyu, cook until
onion is soft. Stir in tomato purée, peanut butter and garlic. Add water
and milk and bring back to the boil, stirring regularly until mixture is
smooth and not too thick. Season with pepper to taste.
   It is important that the consistency is not too thick as it will become
thick and lumpy if overcooked. MAKES 2½ CUPS

AVOCADO AND YOGURT DRESSING   G&Y

1 ripe avocado
½ lemon
400 ml (14 fl oz) yogurt

3 cloves garlic (crushed)
pinch of salt and pepper

Halve the avocado and scoop out the flesh, blend or mash immediately with lemon juice. Fold yogurt and garlic into avocado mixture until smooth. Season to taste, or season with chilli or cayenne pepper. MAKES 2½ CUPS

YOGURT HERB DRESSING   G

125 ml (5 fl oz/½ cup) natural
  yogurt
1 clove garlic, crushed
15 ml (1 tbsp) cider vinegar

5 ml (1 tsp) clear honey
15 g (½ oz) parsley
15 g (½ oz) mixed mint and herbs
pinch of salt and pepper

Place all ingredients except herbs in a bowl, adding salt and pepper to taste and mix thoroughly with a fork. Add herbs finely chopped and mix well or blend for 1–2 minutes. Chill until required. MAKES 1 CUP

CREAMY TOMATO DRESSING   G&Y

30 ml (2 tbsp) home-made
  mayonnaise
1 tomato, chopped

10 ml (2 tsp) lemon juice
2.5 ml (½ tsp) dried or 1 tsp fresh
  basil

Blend all the ingredients together on low speed. MAKES ABOUT ⅓ CUP

OIL AND FRUIT DRESSING   G

30 ml (2 tbsp) olive oil
15 ml (1 tbsp) sesame oil
5 ml (1 tsp) mayonnaise
5 ml (1 tsp) mustard

juice from a lemon or 15 ml (1 tbsp)
  wine vinegar
5 ml (1 tsp) concentrated apple juice
  (optional)
black pepper to taste

Blend all the ingredients together until smooth. This dressing keeps well in the fridge in a sealed container. MAKES 1 CUP

LUNCHES AND DINNERS

GRILLED (BROILED) SARDINES   G&Y

Wash and dry sardines, dust with peppered flour (non-wheat flour for restricted diets) and grill (broil) for 5–10 minutes depending on size, turning once.

or

Place sardines on the grill (broiler), sprinkle with pepper and olive oil and grill for 5–10 minutes depending on size, turning once.

STUFFED PEPPERS   G

1 medium onion
2 sticks celery
100 g (4 oz) mushrooms
1 large tomato
1 medium-sized carrot
25 g (1 oz/½ stick) margarine
100 ml (5 fl oz/½ cup) water
5 ml (1 tsp) tomato purée (paste)

2.5 ml (½ tsp) yeast extract (Miso)
4 medium-size green or red (bell)
  peppers
30 ml (2 tbsp) buckwheat or other
  grain-free flour
seasoning to taste
100 g (4 oz) Cheddar cheese, grated

Chop the onion, celery, mushrooms and tomatoes and dice the carrot, melt margarine and fry onion, carrot, celery and mushrooms together for 5 minutes. Stir in the tomato, water, tomato purée and yeast extract. Cover and simmer for 10–15 minutes, until just tender. Meanwhile, halve peppers lengthways and remove the seeds, then steam for 10 minutes. Arrange in an ovenproof serving dish. Drain vegetables, reserving the cooking liquid. Fill the peppers with the vegetables. Sprinkle the flour into the vegetable liquid and bring to the boil. Adjust seasoning to taste. Pour over the peppers, sprinkle with the cheese and bake in the oven at 200°C (400°F/Mark 6) for 15 minutes. Serve at once. SERVES 4

SPANISH OMELETTE   G&Y

1 small onion, chopped
25 ml (1 fl oz/¼ cup) water
1 stick celery, chopped
1 green (bell) pepper

2 eggs
5 ml (1 tsp) butter
2 tomatoes, chopped
parsley (scissor-snipped)

Place the onions and water in a sealed pan over a medium heat. When water begins to boil reduce the heat to low. Add celery and green pepper and continue cooking until soft. Do not overcook. Beat eggs, melt butter in a medium frying pan over a low heat. Pour in beaten eggs and allow to cook gently. Strain vegetables, tip onto partly cooked omelette and add tomatoes. When cooked serve sprinkled with parsley. SERVES 1

STIR-FRY VEGETABLES   G†*

There are many different combinations of vegetable in season that can be used for stir-frying. You can use six or seven different vegetables or only two or three.

To obtain the best results, stir-fry vegetables should be cooked with the minimum oil at a high heat as rapid cooking seals in the flavour.

Here are some nice last-minute additions to your stir-fry. Experiment to find your favourite seasoning and flavouring. Less well-known ingredients are available from healthfood shops.

*Seasoning

Salt, pepper, chilli, grated ginger, five spice (use very moderately), sesame seeds (ground), fenugreek (ground), turmeric, coriander, paprika, nori seaweed (toasted and crumbled).

*Flavouring

Shoyu/tamari, Miso (all Japanese/Chinese condiments made from soya beans), sesame oil, tahini (sesame seed butter), sunflower oil, safflower oil, sherry, vermouth, lemon juice.

450 g (1 lb) fresh broccoli
225 g (8 oz) cauliflower
15 ml (1 tbsp) oil
2.5 cm (1 in) fresh ginger, sliced and finely shredded
2 large carrots, peeled and sliced

2.5 ml (½ tsp) sesame oil
225 g (8 oz) fresh bean sprouts
225 g (8 oz) Chinese leaves or white cabbage, shredded
2.5 ml (½ tsp) salt

Separate the broccoli heads into small florets and peel and slice the stems. Separate the cauliflower florets and slice stems. Heat oil in a large wok or frying pan. When it is moderately hot add ginger shreds. Stir-fry for a few seconds. Add the carrots, cauliflower and broccoli and stir-fry for 2–3 minutes then add sesame seed oil, bean sprouts and Chinese leaves or white cabbage. Stir-fry for further 2–3 minutes. Season to taste. Serve at once. SERVES 4–6

* † and Y if yeast-free flavouring selected

Ginger can be substituted for garlic and soy sauce can be added in final stage of frying before serving.

MACKEREL WITH HERBS (IN FOIL)   G&Y

4 medium-sized fresh mackerel, gutted
juice of one lemon
freshly ground black pepper

4 small bunches of 4 different fresh mixed herbs, e.g. tarragon, chives, parsley and sage
little olive oil

Preheat oven to 240°C (475°F/Mark 9). Wash mackerel and sprinkle insides with lemon juice. Add generous sprinkling of pepper. Put bunch of mixed herbs inside each fish and brush skin with oil to avoid sticking, wrap each fish individually in foil, quite tightly, bake for 10–12 minutes and serve. SERVES 4

STUFFED MACKEREL IN FOIL

2 large oranges
4 tbsp porridge (rolled oats)
1 medium-sized onion, finely chopped
1 tbsp parsley, finely chopped
1 tbsp raisins

1 apple, grated
pinch of salt
1 tsp dried rosemary or 4 sprigs fresh rosemary
4 medium-sized fresh mackerel, gutted

Grate zest of orange, chop flesh into small pieces, discarding pips and any tough pith. Mix the orange zest and flesh with oats, onion, parsley, raisins and grated apple and pinch of salt. Divide mixture into 4 and stuff mackerel loosely. Place rosemary in each fish. Bake in foil as above for about 40 minutes. SERVES 4

VEGETARIAN GOULASH   G

45 ml (3 tbsp) oil
1 medium onion, sliced
2 medium carrots, diced
2 medium courgettes (zucchini), sliced
½ small white cabbage, finely shredded
15 ml (1 tbsp) paprika

2.5 ml (½ tsp) caraway seeds
2.5 ml (½ tsp) mixed herbs
pinch of nutmeg
600 ml (1 pint) tomato juice
300 ml (½ pint) water
1 vegetable stock cube
142 ml (¼ pint) soured cream or natural yogurt

Heat oil in large saucepan and sauté the onion and carrot until the onion is transparent. Add courgettes and cabbage and cook over medium heat for 10 minutes, stirring frequently. Stir in paprika, caraway seeds, herbs and nutmeg, then add tomato juice, water and stock cube. Cover and simmer for about 20 minutes until the vegetables are just tender. Adjust seasoning with a small pinch salt and pepper. Serve each portion with a drop of soured cream or yogurt. Serve at once. SERVES 4–6

STEAMED FISH (WITH GARLIC, SPRING ONIONS [SCALLIONS] AND GINGER)   G&Y

350 g (12 oz) firm white fish fillets (cod, sole etc)

2.5 ml (½ tsp) salt

15 ml (1 tbsp) fresh ginger, finely chopped

30 ml (2 tbsp) spring onions (scallions), finely chopped

15 ml (1 tbsp) light soy sauce (not for yeast-free diet)

15 ml (1 tbsp) oil, preferably groundnut

5 ml (1 tsp) sesame oil

2 garlic cloves, peeled and thinly sliced

Rub cleaned and dried fish with salt both sides and leave for 30 minutes. Steam fish over simmering water until just cooked, covering steamer tightly. Sprinkle on the ginger, spring onions and light soy sauce. Heat the two oils together in small saucepan, when hot add garlic slices and brown. Pour the garlic oil mixture over the top of the fish. Serve at once. SERVES 4

SNOW PEAS WITH TIGER PRAWNS   G&Y

450 g (1 lb) snow peas (mange tout))

450 g (1 lb) uncooked tiger prawns

375 g (13 oz) uncooked broad oriental rice noodles

5 ml (1 tsp) finely chopped root ginger

45 ml (3 tbsp) sesame oil

30 ml (2 tbsp) oyster sauce

5 ml (1 tsp) sugar

15 ml (1 tbsp) sherry or white wine

fresh coriander to decorate

Top and tail the snow peas and wash them. Clean and wash the prawns and pat them dry with kitchen paper. Place the noodles in boiling water and simmer gently for 3 minutes, until slightly undercooked. Place the ginger and the oil in a wok and heat. Fry the snow peas briefly in the hot oil stirring constantly. Remove and place on a warmed dish. Place the tiger prawns in the wok and cook until they become pink. Drain the noodles and rinse with cold water to remove the starch. Return snow peas to the wok with the prawns, add the oyster sauce and the sugar, and simmer for another minute or two. Gently pour one tablespoon of sherry or white wine around the circumference of the wok, and then remove peas and prawns from the wok with a slatted spoon and transfer to a dish. Place noodles in the wok and quickly stir-fry them in the remaining oil turning constantly. Turn the noodles out onto a flat platter and place the snow peas and prawns on the top. Decorate with fresh coriander and serve immediately. SERVES 4

Variation If you like spicy food, before stir-frying the noodles mix 5 ml (1 tsp) chilli sauce with the hot oil and then place the noodles in the wok.

FRAGRANT LAMB   G&Y

2–3 lb (900 g–1.3 kg) fillet joint of
   leg of lamb or 6 fillets of lamb
45 ml (3 tbsp) sesame oil
1 clove of garlic, chopped
1.25 cm (½ in) lump of root ginger,
   chopped
whole spring onion
45 ml (3 tbsp) light soy sauce

30 ml (2 tbsp) brandy
45 ml (3 tbsp) white wine
black pepper to taste or a sprinkling
   of black peppercorns
5 ml (1 flat tsp) cornflour
8 large lettuce leaves to decorate the
   serving plate
sprig of coriander

Seal the lamb by cooking in a little hot sesame oil for two minutes each side. Remove the lamb from the hot oil and place in a pressure cooker. Add the chopped garlic, chopped ginger, the whole spring onion, the remaining sesame oil, soy sauce, brandy, white wine, and black pepper or peppercorns. Put the lid on the pressure cooker and bring to the boil. Lower the heat, and cook at pressure for 35 minutes. Decorate a large serving dish with lettuce leaves ready to receive the lamb. Remove the pressure cooker from the heat and place under cold running water to cool. Place the lamb on a chopping board and slice into portions. Arrange the chops or the sliced lamb joint on the serving dish and place in the oven to keep warm whilst you prepare the sauce. Drain the juice and thicken with the cornflour, stirring constantly. Remove the serving dish from the oven, pour the sauce over the lamb and decorate with the coriander. Serve immediately. SERVES 6

LAMB PAPRIKA   G

2 onions, sliced
50 g (2 oz) mushrooms, sliced
2 carrots, sliced
4 lamb chops (lean)

30 ml (2 tbsp) paprika
450 ml (¾ pint) water
15 ml (1 tbsp) cornflour (cornstarch)
   (or alternative grain-free flour)

Mix vegetables together and place in casserole. Arrange chops on top. Stir paprika into water and pour over chops, cover and cook until chops are tender. Remove vegetables and chops and arrange on warm serving dish. Mix cornflour with a little cold water and use to thicken liquid from chops. Cook for 2–3 minutes, pour over chops. SERVES 2–4

LIVER WITH ORANGE   G

225 g (8 oz) lamb's liver
30 ml (2 tbsp) wholewheat flour (or
   alternative grain-free flour)
2.5 ml (½ tsp) dried thyme or basil
25 ml (1½ tbsp) sunflower oil

1 orange, peeled and sliced
grated orange peel
15 ml (1 tbsp) soy sauce
30 ml (2 tbsp) orange juice

Wash liver, slice thinly, pat dry with kitchen paper. Cut out and discard stringy pieces, coat in flour seasoned with herbs. Heat oil in a frying pan and fry liver pieces gently for 5 minutes, turning to cook evenly. Add orange slices and peel, soy sauce and orange juice. Heat through gently and serve. SERVES 2

NUT ROAST   G

1 medium onion
25 g (1 oz/¼ stick) butter/margarine
225 g (8 oz/2 cups) mixed nuts
100 g (4 oz/2 cups) cooked brown
   rice

200 ml (½ pint) vegetable stock
10 ml (2 tsp) yeast extract (Miso)
5 ml (1 tsp) mixed herbs
salt and pepper to taste

Chop onions and sauté in butter until transparent. Grind nuts in a blender or food processor until quite fine. Heat stock and yeast extract to boiling point, then combine all the ingredients including the cooked brown rice together and mix well until the mixture is a fairly slack consistency. Turn into greased shallow baking dish, level the surface, and bake in oven at 180°C (350°F/Mark 4) for 30 minutes until golden brown. SERVES 4–6

COLOURFUL LENTILS   G

60 ml (4 tbsp) oil
3 cloves garlic, crushed
4 carrots, chopped
1 green (bell) pepper, chopped
1 red (bell) pepper, chopped
5 ml (1 tsp) basil
3 sticks celery, chopped

15 ml (1 tbsp) brown rice miso
900 ml (1½ pints) hot water
675 g (1½ lb) tomatoes, skinned, seeded and chopped
280 g (10 oz) lentils, not presoaked
30 ml (2 tbsp) chopped parsley
seasoning to taste

Heat oil in a pan and add the garlic, carrots, green and red peppers, basil and celery. Cook until the ingredients are soft. Mix the brown rice miso with hot water and add this to mixture, together with the tomatoes. Stir in the lentils. Season to taste. Simmer for 1 hour. Serve, garnished with the chopped parsley. SERVES 4 OR 6 AS A STARTER

STUFFING FOR ROAST CHICKEN   G

1 stick celery, finely chopped
2 cloves garlic, crushed
30 ml (2 tbsp) sunflower oil
60 g (2 oz/¼ cup) uncooked long grain brown rice
150 ml (¼ pint) hot water

120 g (4 oz/2 cups) mushrooms, sliced
30 g (1 oz/⅙ cup) sultanas
60 g (2 oz/⅓ cup) dried apricots, soaked and chopped
30 ml (2 tbsp) tarragon

Fry the celery and garlic in the oil for 2–3 minutes. Add the rice and sauté for a few minutes. Pour in the hot water, stir, then simmer for 5–6 minutes until most of the water has been absorbed, but the rice is still hard. Remove from the heat and mix in the remaining ingredients. Allow to cool for a little, then use to stuff the chicken.

SWEETS

FRUIT JELLY   G

22 g (¾ oz) gelatine
600 ml (1 pint) unsweetened fruit
  juice
  e.g. apple, pineapple

Sprinkle the gelatine on 1 tbsp heated fruit juice and stir well until dissolved. Add the rest of the juice. Put into a wetted mould and chill until set. SERVES 4

DRIED FRUIT COMPOTE AND YOGURT   G

15 g (½ oz/1 tbsp) sugar
600 ml (1 pint) water
5–10 cm (2–3 in) stick of cinnamon

450 g (1 lb) mixed dried fruit e.g.
apple rings, peaches, apricots,
prunes, pears and sultanas

Dissolve the sugar in the water over a gentle heat, add the cinnamon. Place the dried fruit in a bowl and pour the syrup over. Cover and leave to soak overnight. If the soaked fruit is not tender, replace in the pan and simmer for a few minutes. Serve cold with yogurt. SERVES 4–6

RHUBARB FOOL   G&Y

25 g (1 oz/¼ stick) margarine
225 g (8 oz) rhubarb

12–25 g (½–1 oz) brown sugar
200 ml (7 fl oz) natural yogurt

Melt margarine in a pan. Add rhubarb and sugar and cook until tender. Purée rhubarb and yogurt together in a blender. Chill before serving. SERVES 4

STUFFED BAKED APPLES   G

4 good-sized cooking apples
1 tbsp honey/sugar-free jam

Stuffing suggestions:
Dates, cinnamon, raisins and honey

Core apples and slit skins in a ring round the middle. Stuff with chosen filling and honey. Bake until fruit is tender. Serve hot or cold. SERVES 4

CARROT CAKE G

4 eggs
225 g (8 oz/1 cup) caster (superfine)
 sugar
grated rind of 1 lemon
225 g (8 oz/2 cups) ground almonds

225 g (8 oz) carrots, finely grated
25 ml (1½ tbsp) rice flour
5 ml (1 tsp) wheat-free baking
 powder

Preheat the oven to 180°C (350°F/Mark 4). Separate the eggs. Place yolks, sugar and lemon rind in a bowl or in a blender or food processor and beat together well. Add the almonds and carrots to this mixture. Stir well. Sift the flour and baking powder together then fold into mixture. In another bowl beat the egg whites until they are stiff, then fold them into the mixture. Grease an oblong baking tray 8×12×2 inches (20×30×5 cm). Spread the mixture out in the tray and bake for 45 minutes. Leave to cool in the tray, then cut into slices. MAKES 10 SLICES

BANANA CREAM G

4 medium bananas
15 ml (1 tbsp) lemon juice

400 ml (15 fl oz/2 cups) yogurt
5 ml (1 tsp) honey

Place all ingredients in the blender and blend until creamy. Chill well before serving. SERVES 4

FRUITY CAKES G

100 g (4 oz/1 stick) butter/margarine
100 g (4 oz) unrefined sugar
 (reduced to caster (superfine)
 sugar consistency in a blender or
 food processor)
2 eggs, beaten

200 g (5½ oz) Trufree No 7 self-
 raising (self-rising) flour, or other
 wheat-free flour
100–150 g (4–6 oz/¾–1 cup) mixed
 raisins, currants and sultanas
 (golden raisins)

Cream butter or margarine and sugar till light and fluffy. Add eggs gradually then fold in flour. Stir in mixed dried fruit. Put mixture into individual cake cases and bake at 190°C (375°F/Mark 5) for 15–18 minutes till risen and golden.

Alternatively place all the mixture in a 500 g (1 lb) loaf tin and cook at 180°C (350°F/Mark 4) for 20–25 minutes for a sweet fruit loaf. MAKES 10 CAKES

GINGER BANANAS   G

4 ripe bananas
small amount preserved ginger

25 g (1 oz) flaked almonds

Slice the bananas into individual dishes (one per person). Rinse the syrup from the preserved ginger and chop fairly finely. Sprinkle ginger over the bananas and top with a few almonds. SERVES 4

Variation Mix in a few drops of lemon juice and sprinkle with sunflower seeds.

EGG CUSTARD   G&Y

175 ml (6 fl oz/¾ cup) milk
2 egg yolks
mild honey to taste

a few drops of real vanilla essence
(optional)

Heat the milk to boiling point and add slowly to the well-beaten egg yolks. Return to the pan, preferably a double boiler, and stir over a gentle heat until the mixture thickens slightly. Sweeten to taste with honey and add a few drops of vanilla essence if liked. The custard will thicken as it cools. SERVES 2

CAKES, BISCUITS AND BREAD

BUCKWHEAT AND RICE BREAD

This makes brown bread which is crisp on the outside and soft on the inside.

300 g (12 oz) buckwheat flour
150 g (6 oz) brown rice flour
1½ packets easy yeast
5 ml (1 tsp) sugar
15 ml (1 tbsp) oil

2.5–5 ml (½–1 tbsp) salt
340–360 ml (just over ½ pint)
  hand-hot water
2 500 g (1 lb) loaf tins

Mix together flours and easy yeast. Add sugar, oil and salt and mix to a thick batter with the hand-hot water. Grease and flour the two loaf tins.

Divide mixture between the two loaf tins, cover and leave to rise in a warm place for 20–30 minutes. Bake at 230°C (450°F/Mark 8) for 35–40 minutes. The bread will slightly contract from the side of the tins when it is cooked. Cool for 5 minutes in the tins and then turn out onto a wire rack. MAKES 14 SLICES (7 EACH LOAF)

POTATO AND RICE BREAD

This is a white bread which is delicious when freshly baked, and subsequently makes very nice toast. It tastes rather like crumpets.

250 g (10 oz) potato flour
200 g (8 oz) brown rice flour
1½ packets easy yeast
5 ml (1 tsp) sugar

15 ml (1 tbsp) oil
2.5–5 ml (½–1 tsp) salt
340–360 ml (just over ½ pint)
    hand-hot water
2 500 g (1 lb) loaf tins

Mix together flours and easy yeast. Add sugar, oil and salt and mix to a thick batter with the hand-hot water. Grease and flour the two loaf tins. Divide mixture between the two loaf tins, cover and leave to rise in a warm place for 20–30 minutes. Bake at 230°C (450°F/Mark 8) for 35–40 minutes. The bread will contract slightly from the side of the tins when it is cooked. Cool for 5 minutes in the tins and then turn out on to a wire rack. MAKES 16 SLICES (8 EACH LOAF)

POTATO SHORTBREAD

150 g (6 oz) potato flour
100 g (4 oz) margarine

50 g (2 oz) sugar
75 g (3 oz) ground almonds

Put all ingredients in to a food processor and beat together for 5–6 seconds. Scrape bowl and repeat the process until a ball of dough is formed. Put dough into a greased 7–8 in (17.5–20 cm) round sandwich tin and press down evenly. Mark out portions with a knife, prick all over and bake at 180°C (350°F/Mark 4) for 35–40 minutes. Cut into wedges and cool in tin. MAKES 8 SLICES

APPLE AND CINNAMON CAKE

4 large cooking apples
225 g (8 oz) brown rice flour
4 large eggs
100 g (4 oz) ground almonds
100 g (4 oz) caster sugar
100 g (4 oz) cooking flora
few drops of almond essence to
    flavour

15 ml (1 tbsp) cinnamon

To decorate:

approximately 16 apple slices
7.5 ml (½ tbsp) of cinnamon
15 ml (1 tbsp) of caster sugar

Grease a deep 8 in (20 cm) loose-bottomed circular baking tin. Pre-heat oven to moderate temperature, 150°C (300°F/Mark2). Peel, core and slice the apples and leave to soak in cold water. Place the flour, eggs, ground almonds, caster sugar, cooking flora and almond essence in the bowl of a mixer and beat until light and fluffy. Line the cake tin with approximately 1½ in (3.75 cm) of mixture. Place most of the apples in the tin and sprinkle with sugar and cinnamon. Spread the additional mixture on to the top of the apples and smooth off the top ready for the decoration. Gently push remaining apple slices into the top of the cake in a circle and sprinkle with cinnamon and sugar. Bake in a moderate oven for at least one hour, until cooked through. Cool briefly, then gently ease the cake out of the tin and onto a plate. Serve hot as a pudding or cold as a cake with whipped or pouring cream. MAKES 8 GOOD SIZED SLICES

ALMOND MACAROONS

2 large egg whites
150 g (6 oz) ground almonds

75 g (3 oz) caster sugar
18 almond halves

Put the unbeaten egg whites into a bowl with the ground almonds, and beat well adding the caster sugar 1 tablespoon at a time. Line biscuit trays with greaseproof paper. With moist hands roll the mixture into balls and flatten in the palm of your hand. Lay the flattened biscuits carefully onto the trays and place an almond half in the middle of each biscuit. Bake in a moderate oven at 180°C (350°F/Mark 4) for 25 minutes or until golden brown. Keep in an airtight tin, or freeze. MAKES 18 (9 PORTIONS)

COCONUT PYRAMIDS

4 egg yolks or two whole eggs   juice and rind of half a lemon
75 g (3 oz) caster sugar   250 g (8 oz) dessiccated (dried and shredded) coconut

Beat the egg yolks and sugar until creamy. Stir in the lemon juice, rind and coconut. Form into pyramid shapes, either with your hands or using a moist egg cup, and place on a greased baking tray. Bake at 190°C (375°F/ Mark 5) until the tips are golden brown. Keep in an airtight tin or freeze.
MAKES ABOUT 24 (12 PORTIONS)

18

STRESS OR DISTRESS?

Let's first take a look at the terms stress and distress. In my opinion a certain amount of stress in life gets the adrenaline going and can be both mentally stimulating and healthy. When the pressure rises to the point where it then becomes uncomfortable, you can rest assured that you've hit the band of distress.

Don't ever underestimate the power of distress on your physical and mental well-being. I've seen many a 'strong' person bite the dust when under incredible pressure. The classic case is a person who seems to cope amazingly well with a disaster or a near-tragedy. They sail through the event appearing cool, calm and collected. Then several months later get physically sick or become emotionally unbalanced. It is now understood that stress places extra nutritional demands on the body. And when we are feeling stressed we often don't eat as well as usual, which can make matters worse.

Part of the game is being able to identify the source of stress and admit honestly that you are finding it a strain.

When you are feeling on top of the world physically and mentally your tolerance of problems or particularly difficult situations may be higher. Whereas when you feel below par, extra problems often seem too much to bear.

Many a physical and emotional illness is precipitated by stress. The body's demand for B vitamins increases when under stress. Often, when people have severe problems, their diet suffers and they either eat insufficient food to meet their requirements or indulge in too much junk food and alcohol. You will have seen from Chapter 14 how deficiencies in B vitamins can lead to nervous and mental disorders. Food allergies are also often linked to distressing situations. These can affect the mind and the body. Migraine headaches, irritable bowel syndrome, agoraphobia, diarrhoea, depression, insomnia, nervous tension, mood swings, restlessness, etc. can all result from stress-induced food intolerance.

A PROBLEM SHARED IS A PROBLEM HALVED

There is no need to pretend you aren't suffering: it's far better to talk over your problems and frustrations, and even have a good cry if you feel like it. Crying can be very therapeutic. Once the problem has been talked through, you may find it gets put a little more into perspective. You may suddenly realize how to cope with the situation immediately, or in the long term. Support and reassurance are very comforting: having a friend to lean on at times of great need is a very valuable asset. There is no substitute for plenty of open, honest communication.

Try to stand outside the problem and examine it clearly. This often helps you to see things more clearly. Sometimes, being so involved in a situation means you can't 'see the wood for the trees'.

Most of all, take time out each day to get your attention off the problem. Consciously daydream, if you like, in a quiet room undisturbed, or go for a long country walk and observe the wonders of nature. Discipline yourself to do this regularly. You'll be surprised how therapeutic these activities can be.

HOW STRESS AFFECTS YOUR BODY

Pay attention to your body telling you it's not very happy. Look out for possible weak areas that are more susceptible to tension build-up. For example:

Forehead	Upper back
Face	Lower back
Neck	Hands
Shoulders	Legs

Clenched teeth, grinding teeth at night, headaches and eye strain are all signs of inner stress. Becoming aware of your weaknesses is half the battle. The stresses and strains of life do tend to build up in the body. We are each affected differently. Some people suffer backaches, whilst others get headaches. When the body becomes loaded with tension we tie up our energy to some extent. The energy flows become blocked and as a result symptoms like headaches and abdominal cramps are likely to become worse.

215

You can gently massage any tense areas or have someone do it for you, preferably each day. Also try to spend 10–15 minutes at the end of the day consciously relaxing your muscles, beginning with your face and working your way down to your toes.

A good massage is soothing. Yoga may help and it is easy to practise simple relaxing techniques at home. There are other suggestions to help you through difficult periods. Meditation, autogenic training and physical exercise seem to be beneficial for some people. It's really a question of choosing a method of relaxation which you are happy to practise regularly.

There are certain areas in your life which you might like to examine if you are feeling stressed.

- Have you taken on so many commitments that you aren't able to really enjoy life?

Some people just can't say 'No'. They have good hearts, and little appreciation of their actual working capacity. If you are guilty of this, do sit back and have a good think about it. Make yourself a work schedule and a leisure schedule and stick to it.

- Have you got any goals or aims in life you are pursuing? Having a strong sense of purpose in life is a great asset. Not having a purpose or direction can have repercussions on your mental well-being and subsequently affect your health. Without a desire to achieve something, life often becomes rather boring and meaningless.

- Have you got many unfinished projects on the go, and never seem to get around to finishing any one of them?

Knowing that you should have completed a project and didn't, especially if it's something promised to another, can be stressful. Make a list of any unfinished projects and then assign a regular time each week, to work through them gradually.

- Is your home and/or work environment tidy and in order, or have you allowed things to pile up around you?

It is difficult to thrive or relax properly in an area which is untidy, disordered or dirty. If you feel there is room for improvement, why not have a grand 'sort out' or clean up – I'll bet you feel better afterwards.

- Do you have plenty of interests and activities to pursue in your spare

216

time? It is healthy to maintain a wide variety of interests: perhaps some activities that you like to indulge in yourself, and also activities and interests you can share with other members of your family, friends and pets.

- Do you take regular exercise and set aside relaxation time for yourself? Exercise and relaxation are both extremely valuable pursuits and contribute greatly to health. The next chapter is on the subject of exercise and should help you to work out an activity plan.

19

THE VALUE OF
EXERCISE AND
RELAXATION

I can't emphasize strongly enough how important exercise and relaxation are in maintaining a healthy body. There have been several studies which demonstrated that exercise was a valuable tool in overcoming depression, and the PMS A symptoms of nervous tension, mood swings, irritability and anxiety.

If you don't like structural exercises you should at least take a brisk walk for half an hour a day. Personally I find swimming one of the most stimulating exercises, especially at the start of the day.

Beyond doubt, exercise raises energy levels, and your spirits. On a regular basis, it also speeds up the metabolism of the body. Although you may have to push yourself initially, I assure you it will pay dividends within a short space of time.

The mind and body work closely together. The mental stress of PMS will be reflected in the physical tension in your body. The muscular aches and pains of PMS such as headaches, neck pain and stiff joints, together with the more obvious low backache and abdominal cramps, all work to increase feelings of anxiety and depression. It's hardly surprising that the heart rate increases, as the nervous and physical tension increases, all adding to feelings of being 'wound up'.

Exercise may provide help for PMS sufferers more than just by acting as a general tonic. Recently, it has been shown that the level of a particular brain hormone, beta-endorphin, a hormone associated with a sense of well-being and pain relief, was found to be low in pre-menstrual sufferers in the few days before their period. The levels during the first phase of the menstrual cycle were normal when compared with healthy women who did not have PMS. Beta-endorphin is an important self-produced hormone, which may affect mood and well-being, and also influence the function of other hormones. Its level can be raised by regular and usually prolonged physical exercise. Potentially, it could also be influenced by dietary and nutritional factors.

Thus, regular physical exercise by stimulating the body's natural production of beta-endorphin might help to prevent the dip that occurs pre-menstrually in PMS sufferers. The value of exercise in PMS has been studied in two papers from North America. Both of these report a modest benefit of aerobic exercise on PMS, especially for mental symptoms. Breast tenderness was not helped very much by this approach. My own experience supports this. Other studies have shown that physical exercise can be of value in the treatment of depression.

However, you can have too much exercise as well. Analysis of a large group of sufferers contacting the WNAS revealed that the least symptoms were experienced by those who exercised three or four times per week. Those who exercised every day had as much PMS as other women but with a smaller degree of relief in the week after their period.

GENERAL ADVICE

- It is important to take time off to care for yourself.

- Ensure that exercise and relaxation become part of your daily lifestyle.

- Choose styles of exercise that suit your personality and lifestyle.

- Make an effort to slow down at the critical time and look to ways of calming your mind and body – particularly important if your coordination suffers and you become clumsy.

- Above all, take a programme of exercise that balances the 3 'S's with some 'R' – universally known as:

STRENGTH, STAMINA, SUPPLENESS AND RELAXATION

Taking each of the elements in turn, I have highlighted the important factors.

S for Strength can be described as the maximum force needed by a muscle or group of muscles to overcome a resistance.

In everyday terms this means being able to push, pull, lift, climb and carry without injuring yourself. Strong back and abdominal muscles will help improve your posture and guard you from most lower back pain.

There is another important element of strength to consider and that is:

E for Endurance is the muscle's ability repeatedly to perform or maintain a task for a prolonged period of time.

There is also cardiovascular (heart and blood vessel function) training which partners muscular endurance training. Different forms of activity will improve the endurance qualities of different muscle groups. For example, running will train the leg muscles much more than the upper body and arms, while swimming will emphasize upper body endurance. Both, however, will increase cardiovascular endurance.

S for Stamina simply means being able to keep going; whether you're walking, swimming, running or cycling – and without stopping or becoming tired!

These types of activity are called 'aerobic' because of the increased need for oxygen by the working muscles. Remember, the heart is a muscle too and it needs exercise just as much as your legs or arms. The lungs are used to oxygenate the blood. With regular exercise, the heart and lungs become more efficient. The benefits of aerobic training mean you eventually achieve better results with less effort. Your heart and lungs will have to work less hard in daily life.

Experts disagree as to exactly how much aerobic exercise you need to benefit or gain from the training effect. It will also vary from person to person. A general rule of thumb is to aim for at least 20 minutes about three times a week.

S for Suppleness and flexibility: the ability to move your joints through their full range of movement. In other words, being able to bend, stretch, reach and turn to your fullest. Of all the fitness elements so far, flexibility must rate as the one most likely to affect your everyday life. It also means protecting your muscles and joints from injury and stiffness, as well as improving your circulation, posture and poise.

Improving your range of movement will also help to improve your performance in other activities. Correct stretching, when practised after your exercise session (as well as before), will help to minimize the likelihood of post-exercise soreness.

R for Relaxation is the art of letting go. Knowing how to let go and with confidence, is probably one of the most important elements of health and fitness. The ability to release unnecessary muscular tension and calm the mind is a wonderful resource to call upon. Tension is tiring and unproductive.

For some, exercise itself is a form of relaxation, while others might turn to a hobby or pastime.

Relaxation and breathing go hand in hand. Indeed, improving your breathing patterns during exercise is one of the keys to success. It also engenders a feeling of alertness and readiness to cope.

Over the weeks of a considered programme of exercise you will increase the efficiency of your heart and lung capacity with deeper breathing.

TIPS AND HINTS ON EXERCISING

To really ensure you gain the maximum benefit from your efforts, take a few moments to read the following tips and hints – they make all the difference to how you feel about your exercising.

- Remember, exercise should be fun and something you look forward to.

- It won't be if you push yourself fast and furiously, it will only leave you exhausted, sore and disappointed with your efforts.

- Really listen to your body. Believe it or not, it knows best!

- Take it slowly and gradually for longer-lasting results.

- Take time to work out your fitness aims and objectives – what do you want to achieve from your efforts? Finding and following the right programme for you is as vital as eating the right food.

- Decide which activity, or blend of activities, will suit you and help to realize your aims.

- Mix and match whenever possible. Avoid boredom by choosing from several activities you know that you will enjoy and stick at. Better still, are they convenient and can you enjoy the company of others at the same time?

- Try to combine some of your exercises with fresh air and sunlight, both of which have proven benefit in helping to relieve PMS symptoms.

- Balance is the key to successful exercising. Give upper and lower body the same amount of work and spread the load.

- Don't expect miracles overnight – be patient and persevere!

- Aim for quality of exercise, not quantity – look forward to it and enjoy it.

PRECAUTIONS

Most people do not need a full medical check-up before exercising, but if you answer YES to any of the following questions, or you are over 35 and a 'first timer', it's best to discuss your plans with your doctor.

Have you ever suffered from, or is there a family history of:

Chest pains or pain in the shoulders?
High blood pressure or heart disease?
Chest problems like asthma or bronchitis?
Back pain or joint pains?
Headaches, faintness or feelings of nausea?
Diabetes?
Are you taking any medication?
Are you recovering from illness or recent operations?
Are you very overweight?
Are you pregnant?

If you have a cold or sore throat, give exercise a miss until you feel better. When you do resume, take it slowly and build up to your pre-illness fitness level gradually. If you ever feel pain, dizziness, nausea or undue tiredness whenever or wherever you exercise, STOP immediately. Rest and wait.

Change your position or slacken off the intensity if relevant. Try again. If the complaint persists, stop and seek professional advice.

Posture pointers

- Stand in front of a full-length mirror with feet about hip-width apart and insteps lifted.

- Gently rock back and forth to find your balance and 'centred' position. Body-weight will feel evenly balanced between balls and heels, as well as inner and outer edges of feet.

- Line knees directly over ankles and gently pull up thigh muscles above the knees.

The standing position

Now stand sideways to the mirror. Push your bottom out and see and feel the lower back arch and tummy bulge. Correct this by pulling in the abdominal muscles and tucking the buttocks under you. See and feel the lower back lengthen as the pubic bone (pelvis) tilts up to the ceiling. This is the pelvic tilt.

- Keep hips level and maintain pelvic tilt as you turn to face mirror.

- Lift ribcage up and away from hips.

- Pull shoulders down from ears; keep them level and aligned over ankles.

- Let arms hang loosely.

- Lift head upwards from crown and feel the back of neck lengthen.

- Hold chin at right angle to ground.

- Feel entire spine lengthen.

Run through these posture pointers and the pelvic tilt frequently throughout the day, to maintain alignment and heighten your awareness.

Warm-up

Now you're ready to warm up. Never miss out this section as it prepares your body for the work to follow. Mobilizing and loosening exercises, plus some preliminary stretches, will help to improve your performance and skill by increasing the body temperature. A warm-up also helps to reduce the risk of injury and soreness. About 10 minutes is all most people need. Similarly, 'warm down' at the end of each session – no matter how rushed you are. End with some rhythmical exercises and slow holding stretches that taper down from more demanding ones. A warm-down will induce a feeling of relaxation and well-being. It will also help to reduce the likelihood of post-exercise stiffness and soreness.

Warm up by moving rhythmically for 10 minutes to your favourite piece of music, working from your feet upwards, gradually using your whole body.

During your warm-down, take it easy, hold your stretches and slow down gradually. This will minimize any soreness and stiffness.

Relieve the tension

This section takes a look at specific exercises and steps you can take to release tension associated with PMS, as well as improve posture and awareness.

Deeper breathing will be promoted, as well as relaxation and a feeling of calm.

Shoulders and neck

Tension and tightness generally collect at the base of the neck and across tops of shoulders. They are mostly due to the way we sit and stand, as well as being our natural reaction to stress – we slouch, so the neck collapses and the shoulders hunch. Not a pretty sight and often it leaves us with a headache due to the constriction of blood supply to and from the brain.

Take positive steps to ovecome these problems by loosening shoulders and paying more attention to posture. See posture pointers on page 223.

To start, stand or sit well with the head centred and breathe well as you:

1. Lift both shoulders up, pull them back and strongly down. Repeat several times.

Tip – Make sure you really squeeze into the upper back and keep chin held in.

224

2. Clasp hands loosely behind lower back and rest them just above buttocks.

Keep elbows bent and hands resting on body throughout.

Squeeze between the shoulder blades so the elbows draw together.

Hold and release slowly.

Repeat several times.

Feel the squeeze between the shoulder blades and the stretch across the chest.

Tip – Keep the shoulders down, head centred and lower back straight.

3. Turn head slowly to look over right shoulder while maintaining length in the neck and keeping shoulders still.

Return to centre and repeat to opposite side.

Repeat several times.

Return to centre and pull chin in to lengthen back of neck.

Tilt head slowly to right shoulder while keeping shoulders level.

Feel the stretch on the opposite side.

Return slowly to centre.

Tip – As you tilt head, imagine you are looking into a mirror to see both cheeks evenly.

Finally, return to centre, pull shoulders down and tuck chin in.

Tilt head gently forwards.

Feel the stretch along the neck.

Return to centre and repeat once more, breathing well.

225

Back and hips

1. Back strengthener

Lie on your front on either a mat or rug, with legs together, forehead on floor and chin tucked in.

Clasp hands loosely and rest them on lower back.

As you breathe out, contract abdominal and buttock muscles and squeeze between the shoulder blades.

Straighten arms down towards your feet and raise chest, shoulders and forehead off the floor to form one continuous line.

Lower slowly to the floor and repeat once more.

2. Back release

From the previous exercise, place hands under shoulders and gently push up onto your knees to lower your bottom back onto your heels.

Fold your body forwards to rest chest on thighs.

Tuck your head down and rest arms down by sides of body.

Tip – If you feel claustrophobic, stretch your arms out in front of you and rest forehead lightly on floor.

3. Pelvic tilt

Use the pelvic tilt as a back release as well as a preliminary movement to abdominal strengtheners.

Pelvic tilts can be done standing, sitting or lying. Take time to practise the movement, as getting it right makes all the difference to the safety and effectiveness of your exercising and alignment.

Start by lying back on a mat or rug.

Bend knees with feet hip-width apart and lengthen back of neck by tucking chin in.

226

As you breathe out, press lower back down on to mat and pull in abdominal muscles.

Feel the pubic bone tilt up to the ceiling and the lower back flatten down against the floor.

Practise several times until you feel confident of the movement.

4. Curl-overs to strengthen abdominal muscles

Strong abdominal muscles help prevent some lower back pain.

Start as for the pelvic tilt and rest hands on your thighs.

As you breathe out, pelvic tilt and curl head and shoulders slowly off the floor, sliding hands towards knees.

Hold for count of four with waist and lower back on floor.

Lie back slowly and repeat four times.

Let go!

Having the ability to release tension and calm the mind is a wonderful resource to call upon. Tension is tiring and wasteful. Knowing how to cope and apply positive resources is the key to successful relaxation. Adopt any position you find comfortable and supportive for your lower back and neck. It may mean sitting in a high-back chair, or lying back with neck supported by a cushion and legs resting on a chair or stool.

Use your breathing to enhance your relaxation and let your restorative side take over.

Remember to pull the shoulders well down from the ears and let arms rest heavily.

Take several deep breaths, feeling the ribcage move up and out like bellows as you breathe in, and downwards as you breathe out.

Your breathing will gradually become more rhythmical as you start to let go.

Run down your body and check where you feel tight.

Are your shoulders up round your ears? Pull them down. Are your hands clenched? Stretch them out and let the fingers curl.

What about your buttocks and lower back? Make an extra effort to relax and release – try the pelvic tilt to prevent back aching.

Concentrate on your legs, particularly ankles and feet. Let them go and feel the whole body soften.

Finally pay attention to your mouth and face. Soften the jaw and let the softness spread over your face – around the nostrils, between and over your eyes and across your forehead to your hairline.

Spend a few quiet moments with yourself.

When you feel ready, take a few deep breaths, have a good stretch and yawn before curling over to one side and sitting up slowly.

20

OTHER VALUABLE THERAPIES

As well as dealing with symptoms on a nutritional level it is important to make sure that your whole body is functioning at optimum level. The years during which you may have suffered nutritional deficiencies, while coping with stressful situations and pre-menstrual symptoms, may well have taken their toll on your body. The body is a very complicated, but delicate network of bones, muscles, ligaments, nerves, organs and blood vessels. Physical symptoms and nervous tension can affect the smooth running of the body processes. When you make a start on your nutritional programme, if your symptoms are intense, you might consider the value of osteopathy, cranial osteopathy, acupuncture, or acupressure. They are powerful tools and can help to bring about speedy relief of symptoms.

OSTEOPATHY

It is not uncommon, through the wear and tear of everyday life, for subtle back or neck problems to occur. I have seen many resistant, long-standing headaches cured by some good osteopathic manipulation. It is certainly worth having a check-up with a qualified osteopath if you feel tension building up in your back or neck, or if you suffer regular headaches.

Cranial osteopathy, or cranio-sacral therapy as it is known, is a specialized form of osteopathy. Unlike conventional osteopathy, it is a gentle yet potent form of therapy. The aim is gently to coax the muscles, tendons, joints and connective tissue to establish correct functions and release restrictions, thus restoring normal circulation, flow of energy and glandular secretions.

The cranio-sacral mechanism is comprised of the cranium (the skull), the sacrum (the bone at the base of the spine), the membranes surrounding the brain, the spinal cord and the fascia of continuous, clingfilm-like sheet that surrounds the muscles, organs, joints and bones. The tension of this fascia, the clingfilm-like lining, is all important. If you have ever worn an all-in-one pants suit that is too tight or too short in the body, you will have experienced some discomfort. If the tension in the body's fascia becomes too tight, you can't just take it off like an uncomfortable piece of clothing, and it is possible that body functions can be affected in the long term.

Cranial osteopaths claim a good success rate with women who have PMS and other menstrual disorders. You will find it very gentle treatment. Here are some experiences of a cranial osteopath who regularly treats women with PMS and menstrual problems. As well as her treatment she recommends that her patients take regular exercise and seek nutritional advice.

Case history 1

The patient experienced migraine and PMS for five to six days prior to each period. She had some lower back strain, reduced mobility in her upper neck and some pelvic congestion. Her neck was treated and normal function restored. As a result, the congestion and strain within the skull were reduced, the migraines were instantly alleviated, and the PMS symptoms reduced. The patient then received nutritional advice and her PMS reduced further.

Case history 2

This patient was a woman aged 44 who suffered with severe PMS, and backache before and during her period. She was very tall and had poor posture. When examined, she had restricted movement in the lower back and pelvic congestion. After treatment over a period of two months she became 90 per cent better.

It is certainly worth finding a local practitioner if you feel the need is there. (See page 254.)

230

ACUPUNCTURE AND ACUPRESSURE

It is worth mentioning the contribution made by traditional Chinese medicine in the treatment of female health problems. According to the severity of the problem, there are two levels at which treatment can be taken. The first level is appropriate for severe symptoms and involves consulting an acupuncturist. Many of the problems mentioned, including PMS, painful periods, irregular periods, fluid retention and distension, pelvic inflammation, migraines, backache, morning sickness and other troubles of pregnancy, menopausal symptoms, depression, anxiety and insomnia may all respond to treatment by acupuncture. If you feel your complaint is too serious or persistent to cope with by yourself, acupuncture is worth considering as a possible option.

Of course you should always ensure that you get help from a properly trained and registered practitioner. You can usually obtain information from your public library or Citizens Advice Bureau. A register is published by the Council for Acupuncture, listing all members of the four recognized and affiliated professional bodies.

As we are concentrating on aspects of self-help, it is worth considering a second level of treatment, more appropriate to the minor or occasional problems which you can sometimes alleviate by self-assessment and treatment at home. This can be done through Shiatsu, the Japanese finger pressure method (sometimes called acupressure). In this system the body is influenced in various ways by stimulating key points, found along the course of energy channels circulating near the skin surface. These are the same as acupuncture meridians, but the points are stimulated by pressure rather than needles.

For Shiatsu to be effective it is important to give the right kind of pressure, for an appropriate length of time. It is no good pushing pressure points like 'magic buttons' and it is important to recognize by the feel whether what you are doing is correct. Provided you adopt the right approach, Shiatsu may be very helpful, whether you enlist the help of a friend or perform it on your own (self-Shiatsu).

Here is a summary of the method and a description of how to find just a few of the most useful points for some of the troubles mentioned.

Pre-menstrual depression/anxiety

First, try working along the inner leg. Also, two inches above the wrist, in between the tendons at the centre of the inner arm, there is a good point to press firmly. Breathing is very important to get your energy flowing smoothly, so try this simple exercise. Kneel on a cushion or carpeted floor and join your hands together with the fingers back to back while pointing the fingertips towards your own upper abdomen. Let your relaxed fingers press into the centre, below the ribs but above the navel. As you do this lean gently forward and exhale. The pressure should lend a little force to the exhalation. Wait for the inhalation to come naturally and raise yourself back again to the upright kneeling position while breathing in. Go gently at first, repeating the action with every breath, leaning a bit further on to your fingers each time. The abdominal muscles may seem tight or tender but try to relax fully at the end of each breath while leaning forward. Only do this 10 times. You may move your fingers up and down or a little way along the ribs to explore for any tension. Afterwards sit quietly for a minute. You may feel like a good stretch before getting up.

Insomnia/headaches

Work with your own fingertips along the base of the skull behind the head where it joins the neck. Feel for any sensitive hollows where the muscles meet the bony ridge and, leaning your head back, let your fingers penetrate and hold for a few breaths. (If you do this for a friend, support her forehead with one hand and use your other hand to find points with finger and thumb on either side of her neck, pressing inward and upward.) For frontal headaches lean forward, letting your fingertips support the forehead just below the eyebrows – it may feel tender, but breathe and relax for several seconds. Also, work generally along the inside edges and soles of the feet, pressing especially around the inside ankle area. Another useful point for headaches can be found by pressing hard into the fleshy area between your finger and thumb – press towards the edge of the bone on the forefinger side.

Period pains

Get comfortable. Feel for sensitive points along the inside of the lower leg between the edge of the bone and the calf muscle. Hold any points with sustained thumb-pressure to the limit of comfort for five or six seconds or longer. You should try to breathe easily in a relaxed way and maintain the pressure until the sensation diminishes a little. To make it easier, reinforce one thumb with the other while pressing. Ask a friend or partner to lean with their thumbs into the area of the sacrum (triangular bony part at the base of your spine between the buttocks), they could explore a little way each side of centre, pressing firmly but gently any tender spots they find (you should say if it is too strong).

If this approach really interests you, there are two particularly good books you could read which are mentioned on the Reading List on page 251. You could also look for Shiatsu classes in your area. If you do not know of any, write to the secretary of the Shiatsu Society whose address is listed in Appendix 5 at the back of the book, page 254. The Society will send you a list of qualified teachers.

Whatever you do, it is important to ensure that you put yourself in the hands of a qualified practitioner. These days all the recognized alternative therapies have official associations. These bodies keep registers of qualified practitioners. It is best to check up as there are, sadly, quite a few non-qualified practitioners who are not to be recommended.

21

OTHER
RELATED PROBLEMS

By now you should have a good idea of what may be causing your pre-
menstrual symptoms and how you can treat them successfully by changing
your diet, taking some nutritional supplements and doing some moderate
exercise. Very often PMS exists together with other health problems. This
may be by chance, but sometimes there is a dietary connection. In this
chapter I want to take a brief look at some common health problems and
situations that can occur alongside PMS.

PAINFUL PERIODS

Painful periods are particularly common in young women, especially
before they start child-bearing. Period pains are not actually part of PMS,
and anyone who experiences severe pain should check with their doctor as
there may be an underlying problem such as fibroids in the womb or ovarian cysts.

Often, however, there is no problem with the anatomy and you may
need to try some self-help measures. There are various options available,
from pain-killers to more natural remedies.

Aspirin, paracetamol and ibuprofen can all be effective, and another
pain-killer that I referred to earlier, mefenamic acid, may also help associated PMS. This pain-killer is only available from your doctor.

A more natural treatment which can sometimes be helpful is the
mineral magnesium, according to one small study from France. This is
worth considering in view of the benefit that magnesium can bring to PMS

as well. Also, changing your diet, taking other supplements and regular exercise might improve your body's chemistry in a way that reduces the level of chemicals that are associated with painful periods. Practically all the women who have been through our programme, who had painful periods initially, noticed that their period pain disappeared.

Heat is helpful, too, as it helps to relax the muscles. The WNAS has discovered a wonderful thermal heat pad that tucks inside your clothes, and helps to soothe away the pain. These pads are especially comforting in winter, and are available by mail order from the WNAS (see page 254).

HEAVY PERIODS

Excessive loss of blood is a problem for up to 10 per cent of menstruating women and is the main factor that leads to iron deficiency and anaemia in women of child-bearing age. Periods tend to get a little heavier with increasing age and with increasing weight, but there are other factors too. It is quite difficult for women to judge accurately just how heavy their periods are, so if your periods seem heavy it would be useful for you to have a blood test to check for anaemia or mild iron deficiency. A serum ferritin test is often the best as it detects low iron stores more accurately than the haemoglobin test.

It is also wise to have a check for gynaecological abnormality, but more often than not none will be found. If you are contemplating the oral contraceptive pill as a means of contraception, you are likely to find that it lessens the menstrual flow. Having said that, we have a great deal of success with regulating the timing and the flow of periods just by improving each individual's nutritional state.

Eating a healthy diet rich in iron and B vitamins, losing weight if you are overweight, and taking specific nutritional supplements is certainly worth a try.

IRREGULAR PERIODS

Irregular periods, especially those that are infrequent, can either be due to being too thin, or can occur in association with being overweight and developing excessive hair growth. This latter situation can be due to cysts on the ovaries (polycystic ovaries), a condition which results in hormone imbalances and can aggravate PMS.

Though polycystic ovaries can be treated by powerful hormonal drugs, they have been shown recently to respond extremely well to a weight-reducing low-fat diet. By losing only a stone in weight, the periods can become more regular, and there can be a reduction in excessive body and facial hair and an improved chance of becoming pregnant.

Being underweight due to illness or a poor diet, as in anorexia nervosa, can also result in irregular or absent periods. This is particularly likely to lead to a serious fall in the level of oestrogen and as a result premature thinning of the bones – osteoporosis. This process can be further accelerated if there is also an excessive amount of exercise, as in some performance athletes or ballet dancers.

PREGNANCY

This is still the best treatment for PMS! But, alas, is not the solution. However, a sound nutritional state during pregnancy is of paramount importance, and it therefore deserves a mention.

Since December 1992 the recommendation of the Chief Medical Officer of the Department of Health in the United Kingdom has been that all women who are intending to become pregnant or who are likely to should eat a healthy diet *before* they conceive. This is to ensure that they receive enough Folic acid, one of the B group vitamins, adequacy of which helps guard against the risks of spina bifida or other damage to the brain and nervous system. If the prospective mother is not eating a diet rich in Folic acid, i.e. fresh vegetables, fruit, oranges, orange juice and fortified breakfast cereals, then she should take a supplement providing 400 mcg per day.

Conversely, too much vitamin A may lead to other problems in pregnancy. Consequently, pregnant women are also advised not to take any vitamin preparations containing animal vitamin A-retinol or to eat liver, which may contain particularly large amounts of this nutrient. This means that if you are taking multi-vitamins, cod liver oil or Optivite you should stop these if you become pregnant. Do not exceed the recommended amount for these or any other vitamin preparations. The risk from excess vitamin A in tablets is mainly theoretical, but that provided by a single serving of liver is many times that to be found in the usual dosage of most vitamins.

POST-NATAL DEPRESSION

The association between depression after childbirth and pre-menstrual problems has been known for many years and was used as evidence that both conditions were due to a lack of the hormone progesterone. This has proved not to be the case in PMS. There is evidence that both conditions may reflect a vulnerability of the body to hormonal changes, and that the ability to tolerate this may in turn be due to both nutritional and social factors. For example, there is now good evidence that post-natal depression is more likely to occur in women with a history of depression or who lack adequate social support to cope with a new-born babe.

Some workers have related post-natal depression to changes in blood calcium or a lack of vitamin B. A healthy diet, plenty of rest, sleep and a supportive and loving environment seem to be good treatment for both post-natal depression and PMS. It is noteworthy that during pregnancy and whilst breastfeeding, the demands for calcium, magnesium and the B vitamins are very high and a lack of most of these can cause changes in mood.

During pregnancy and breastfeeding, the good nutrients go sailing across the placenta or out through the breast milk to the baby. If the nutrients are not replaced in adequate quantities it stands to reason that at the end of the day it is the mother who will end up a depleted heap! I often hear from mothers who suddenly develop severe PMS symptoms after pregnancy or breastfeeding, especially after the birth of a second child, which often seems to be the straw that breaks the camel's back.

STERILIZATION

Female sterilization is most often achieved by cutting or clipping the Fallopian tubes that normally carry the eggs released from the ovary to the womb. By preventing the union between the egg and the sperm a high degree of protection against pregnancy is achieved. The operation, which is usually performed under general anaesthetic, can cause a few minor changes in hormone balance but these usually settle down within six months. Though it is not officially recognized as being a factor in the production of PMS, my experience is that for a few women it appeared to be an important and unwelcome influence as borne out by Jane's testimony.

'Ever since I was sterilized I had PMS symptoms. I never had any kind of PMS or period problems before. I went back to the doctor who sterilized me when I started to get these symptoms every month. He just turned around and said, "You women are all the same. You don't want any more babies, we sterilize you and then you come back and complain."

The doctor assured me that sterilization had nothing to do with the symptoms I was getting now, but I insisted that before the sterilization I *had felt perfectly OK, terrific every month and did not have any PMS symptoms whatsoever. I was very annoyed by his reaction.'*

Why symptoms suddenly arrive is not really understood, although it is believed progesterone levels drop for a while after sterilization. However, we have managed to eliminate the symptoms once again with the nutritional programme. Obviously, much more research is needed into the whole issue of the implications of nutritional deficiencies.

THE MENOPAUSE

For most women, PMS should be diminishing at the time of the menopause. This is certainly true for many, as numerous surveys have shown that the peak age for experiencing PMS symptoms is mid-thirties with a fall off thereafter. However, for some women PMS symptoms may worsen as the menopause approaches, and the two can blend together. The symptoms are quite different. At the menopause, which is characterized by the cessation of periods, there are symptoms of oestrogen deficiency such as vaginal dryness and shrinkage of breast tissue. The hot flushes and sweats are due to surges of other hormones from the pituitary gland at the base of the brain which is trying to persuade the failing ovaries to carry on working. Again, as in menstruation itself or post-delivery, there is considerable variation in individual women's ability to tolerate these hormonal changes.

Associated symptoms such as depression, mood changes, weight gain, fatigue and insomnia are not characteristic of the menopause, but do genuinely appear more frequent at this time. Changing your diet as if to combat PMS is as effective at this time of life. Magnesium and the essential fatty acids appear to be important in the normal functioning of the ovaries. Making sure that there is an adequate supply of these and other nutrients may help ease the passage of menopausal symptoms.

Interestingly, in the Orient menopausal symptoms are less of a problem than they are in the West, and this has been attributed to the effects on hormone metabolism of a diet low in fat, high in fibre and plentiful in fresh fruit and vegetables.

Thinning of the bones leading to osteoporosis is particularly likely to accelerate around menopause with the loss of protective oestrogen. Calcium and exercise can limit this process and a specialized supplement rich in magnesium and multi-vitamins, Gynovite, may also help improve bone density. Many women are unable to take hormone replacement therapy (HRT), either for medical reasons, or because they experience side-effects. For example, it is thought that one-third of women on HRT experience symptoms of PMS, and of course they continue to have a monthly bleed. For the last eight years the WNAS has been providing a programme for women experiencing menopausal symptoms with a great deal of success.

Hormone replacement therapy has become very popular in the US and is being greeted with much enthusiasm in many quarters of the UK. It can be taken in the form of pills similar to oral contraceptives, as an implant inserted under the skin or as a patch applied to the skin of the abdomen or buttock. Some women swear by it, and others cannot tolerate it, so there has to be a natural alternative.

In my experience over the last 10 years, finding the right diet to suit your body, taking specific nutritional supplements in the short term and moderate regular exercise can only serve to improve your general well-being. Once you have learned what your body requires, not only do you stand a good chance of overcoming your symptoms, but you will be far more likely to improve your quality of life, and improve your chances of avoiding the illnesses that can occur later in life, like heart disease, mental illness, or cancer.

22

MEN WHO NO LONGER SUFFER

I didn't feel that the book would be complete without giving a voice to the men in our lives. I have concentrated so far on how women suffer with PMS. But it's not just women who suffer, let's face it, the men are very definitely on the receiving end! Women who have supportive partners have a far easier time on the programme than those whose partners refuse to acknowledge the condition and instead of being understanding, just simply fight back and turn off.

I have had the good fortune to hear from many men who were deeply concerned about the welfare of their women, once they understood that PMS was a real condition, which would respond to treatment.

I think it's important for women to stand back and examine some of the viewpoints, in retrospect, of men who have lived with PMS sufferers before, during and after their nutritional programme. I'm happy to say they can mostly look back and laugh, probably with relief, for the storm is over.

Tom Moor, Jane's husband, is relieved to say that he got back the girl he married.

'Jane was very irritable, she couldn't hold a conversation without snapping. I couldn't touch her for two weeks before her periods as her breasts were so sore and tender. She rarely wanted to go out and would make excuses to stay at home. When she had PMS she changed from being very happy-go-lucky to being bitchy, irritable and tired.

When she was pre-menstrual I used to keep out of her way. I still showed her that I loved her and waited patiently for her one good week each month. We were hoping for an early menopause.

The nutritional programme has made a tremendous difference to our lives. We are able to lead a normal life again. My wife laughs and jokes and she is popular at work.

My advice to other men is to seek help as it is available. Once their partner is on a nutritional programme, help her to persevere, as it will pay dividends in the long run. I feel that more education for men is necessary, more widespread information directed at couples. I, like most men, was totally baffled as to what the cause of the problem was.'

Don, June Garson's husband couldn't imagine what the consequences might have been had she not received help.

'Generally speaking I am a calm, tolerant person. I tried to make allowances, but I didn't understand the problem. It was like living with a "time bomb" not knowing when it was going to go off! June was permanently "uptight" and tearful pre-menstrually. She was unable to cope with life or deal with the children rationally.

Once on the nutritional programme an immediate improvement was noticeable. Her new-found state of mind and feeling of well-being turned the clock back to the time when we met, prior to our children being born. She reverted back personality-wise to the girl I fell for. I no longer dread the time of the month.

My advice to other men is as follows:

Be totally committed to discussing the subject in detail with your partner, read extensively on the subject and INSIST on her seeking help, not only for her sake, but for the rest of the family. Ignorance of the subject is the major hurdle to overcome.

I found your literature and your "cure" very interesting as I employ 150 people, many of them women. As a result of my experience with my wife I was able to realize that a staff problem affecting many employees was due to the PMS of a particular female employee. I have been able to discuss her problem sympathetically and we hope to solve the unrest in the office, as on my recommendation she has written to you for your help.'

Nadine's boyfriend felt that the biggest change for him was that he no longer had to duck to avoid the flying saucepans!

'Nadine's hysterical and often violent acts of throwing objects did cause anger, but more usefully, it improved my reaction time and my catching abilities no end!'

Life was difficult to cope with for Nadine. There were times of great frustration when new remedies for PMS failed to work. Since introducing the nutritional programme into her life, the quality of life for Nadine and her partner has increased enormously.

'I think the key to coping with PMS is to be patient and caring. If her irritability makes you irritable, then feel it, but don't show it. If her hysteria is frightening then allow yourself to be afraid, but be bigger than your fear, and calm her down. Be practical, do the cooking or take over the task she is finding difficult to cope with. Give up your time because you can bet she's feeling worse than you've ever done, and deserves your understanding and a shoulder to lean on. Tell her you love her and reassure her, and most of all, mean it.'

This bittersweet excerpt is from a letter written by the husband of one of our patients:

'I am Dodd, a roofing contractor with eight children and a wife with severe PMS symptoms. She was a complete Jekyll and Hyde character when her PMS struck.

Knowing what divorce can do to a family, I had to have the patience of Job with Eleanor. But after violent attacks (both on myself and the children), outrageous outbursts, locking herself into hotel rooms, insults, screams of rage, alienation from reality, a suicide attempt, and jealous

242

behaviour I had had it. Bearing in mind that for most of the month she was warm, affectionate and everything a wife should be.

The worst of it all was after an attack when the illness had left her and she would creep back to me. Then I had to play the part of the caring husband again.

How can you expect a young couple with two children to come to terms with this terrible PMS problem when there is nowhere to go, nobody to see them? PMS is a dreadful affliction. It is self-destructive, life-threatening and family-life threatening. When I was a child, I would go to see a horror film and on it would be a pit of snakes – provided you did not disturb them they left you alone but woe betide you if you disturbed them. It was the same with Eleanor if she stuck to the diet or went on a binge.

Women are such beautiful creatures, advanced both mentally and physically from the male. More adaptable, stronger, philosophical, and yet they have to cope with some of the most awful female problems. Is this the price a woman has to pay for her beauty?

Eleanor is now cured of her PMS symptoms. I know she is cured and the WNAS has been responsible. The reason (after trying everything else) I know they have hit the nail on the head is because if complacency sets in and she starts pinching sweets, eating curries and drinking, I can guarantee by the end of her monthly cycle she will be going through agony. I am eternally grateful.'

His advice to other men is as follows:

1. A woman has to realize that she has a problem and that it is not everybody else around her that is wrong, but herself.

2. If and when she realizes this, she is 49% there.

3. She has to get the husband to realize (buy him a dummy to suck; he will need it to bite hard on). You are then 98% there.

4. The last 2% is really just the beginning. When it has been realized, you still have an awful long way to go. But it is like everything else in life, you do not get owt for nowt. This now is when you really have to work hard. It is just like any other illness – if left untreated, it just gets worse.

Isn't that great? What wonderful understanding! The common factor for most men who are supportive, seems to be that they were educated on the subject of PMS. When they don't understand what's going on, they obviously find it more difficult to be supportive in the long term, which is quite understandable.

On behalf of PMS sufferers I would like to thank the supportive men of the world for being willing to share the problem. With more education, communication and understanding in the future on the subject of PMS, far fewer lives will be needlessly disrupted.

1 DICTIONARY OF TERMS

Abbreviations used

g = gram, mg = milligram (100 mg = 1 g), mcg = microgram (100 mcg = 1 mg), iu = international unit, kj = kilojoule

ADRENAL GLANDS. The adrenal glands are two small glands situated at the top of the kidneys. They produce several different hormones, most of which are steroid hormones. Hormones from the adrenal glands influence the metabolism of sugar, salt and water and several other functions.

ALDACTONE. This is a diuretic drug which helps fluid retention. It inhibits the action of aldosterone, a hormone from the adrenal glands. It is also known as spironolactone.

ALDOSTERONE. This is a steroid hormone produced by the adrenal glands which is involved in salt and water balance. When it is produced in excess it causes the body to hold water and sodium salt.

ALLERGY. An unusual and unexpected sensitivity to a particular substance which causes an adverse reaction. Foods, chemicals and environmental pollutants are common irritants and they may cause a whole range of symptoms including headaches, abdominal bloating and discomfort, skin rashes, eczema and asthma.

AMENORRHOEA. A complete absence of periods.

AMINO ACIDS. Chains of building blocks which combine together to form the proteins that make living things. There are some 20 or more amino acids, some of which are essential and some non-essential.

ANTI-DEPRESSANTS. These are drugs used to suppress symptoms of depression.

BROMOCRIPTINE. A powerful drug, used to suppress the hormone prolactin. Further details of this can be found in Chapter 12, on conventional remedies. It is occasionally used in the treatment of PMS.

CARBOHYDRATES. Carbohydrates are the main source of calories (kjs) in almost all diets. *Complex carbohydrates* are essential nutrients and occur in the form of fruits, vegetables, pulses and grains. They are important energy-giving foods. There are two sorts of complex carbohydrates: the first are digestible, such as the starches, and the second are not digestible and are more commonly known as 'fibre'.
Refined carbohydrates. These consist of foods that have been processed and refined. White or brown sugar and white flour have, in the process of refining, had many of the vitamins and minerals present in the original plant removed. Further details on this may be found in Chapter 11.

CERVIX. The neck of the womb which projects downwards into the vagina.

CORPUS LUTEUM. Literally, a little yellow gland or body. It is the part of the ovary that remains after the egg has left. It produces two hormones, oestrogen and progesterone, during the second half of the menstrual cycle.

DAY 1 OF CYCLE. The first day of the menstrual bleeding, the day the period arrives, is the first day of the menstrual cycle.

246

DEFICIENCY. A lack of an essential substance, e.g. a vitamin.

DIURETICS. Drugs which cause an increased production of urine by the kidneys. They are used to treat fluid retention.

DOPAMINE. Dopamine is a brain chemical affecting mood. It has a sedating effect.

DYSMENORRHOEA. This is a term used to describe pain occurring during periods.

ENDOCRINE GLANDS. Glands that secrete hormones and regulate other organs in the body. The thyroid and the pituitary glands are endocrine glands.

ENDOMETRIOSIS. A condition in which the lining of the uterus begins to grow outside the uterus in the abdominal cavity. It is usually a painful condition and can be a cause of infertility.

ENDORPHINS. Hormones from the pituitary gland and fluid in the spine which are believed to help control moods, behaviour and part of the workings of the pituitary gland itself. They may also have an effect on how sugar is used in the body, and on other amounts of hormones released from the pituitary gland and the ovaries. If this is so, the production of oestrogen and progesterone could be affected by endorphins.

ESSENTIAL FATTY ACIDS. One of the essential groups of foods which we need to eat to remain healthy. These are essential fats that are necessary for normal cell structure and body function. There are two: linoleic and linolenic acids. They are called 'essential' as they cannot be made by the body but have to be eaten in the diet.

FALLOPIAN TUBES. A pair of slender tubes through which the egg passes on its way from the ovary to the uterus. Fertilization occurs in the Fallopian tubes. Very rarely the egg remains in the tube and grows: this is called an ectopic pregnancy, and is a medical emergency accompanied by severe abdominal pain.

FOLLICLE. A small sac in the ovary containing an egg (ovum). After release of the egg at mid cycle the follicle becomes a corpus luteum.

FOLLICLE STIMULATING HORMONE (FSH). A hormone of the pituitary gland which stimulates the growth of the follicles in the ovaries.

FOLLICULAR PHASE. The first half of the menstrual cycle when an egg is growing in the ovary. The egg is surrounded by cells which produce the hormone oestrogen and which thus prepares the uterus for conception. The egg and surrounding cells are called a follicle.

GLUCOSE. A form of sugar, found in the diet or released by the liver into the bloodstream, which is then used by the brain for energy. This is the only source of energy usable by the brain.

GRAAFIAN FOLLICLE. A mature egg which is surrounded by a bag of fluid within the ovary.

HORMONES. Substances formed chiefly in the endocrine glands, which then enter the bloodstream and control the activity of an organ or body function. Adrenaline and insulin are hormones, as are oestrogen and progesterone.

HYPERHYDRATION – too much water present. This is a term used to describe water retention in the body.

HYPOGLYCAEMIA – LOW BLOOD SUGAR. This is a condition in which there is a deficiency of glucose in the bloodstream, often caused by an excess of insulin or a lack of food. As glucose is required for normal brain function, mental disturbance can occur as can other symptoms: headaches, weakness, faintness, irritability, palpitations, mood swings, sweating and hunger. One of the commonest contributing factors is an excess of refined carbohydrates in the diet.

HYPOTHALAMUS. The region of the brain controlling temperature, hunger, thirst and the hormones produced by the pituitary gland.

HYSTERECTOMY. A surgical procedure to remove the womb and the Fallopian tubes. Sometimes one or more ovaries are also removed.

LUTEAL PHASE. The time after the egg has left the follicle in the ovary, and the follicle then becomes a gland known as the corpus luteum. The corpus luteum produces progesterone.

LUTEINIZING HORMONE (LH). The pituitary hormone which fosters the development of the corpus luteum.

MENORRHAGIA. An excessive loss of blood during each period.

MENSES. The discharge of blood and tissue lining from the uterus, which occurs approximately every four weeks between puberty and the menopause.

MENSTRUAL CYCLE. The monthly cycle involving the pituitary gland, ovaries and uterus in which an egg is produced ready for conception to take place. In each cycle an egg in the ovary is released and the lining of the womb develops ready for conception and implantation of the fertilized egg. If this does not occur, the lining of the womb is shed and a period occurs.

MENSTRUAL SYMPTOMATOLOGY DIARY. A chart which is a daily record of all symptoms that occur throughout the menstrual cycle.

METABOLISM. The process by which the body maintains life. It is the cycle of nutrients being broken down to produce energy, which is then used by the body to build up new cells and tissues, provide heat, growth, and physical activity. The metabolic rate tends to vary from person to person, depending on their age, sex and lifestyle.

MITTELSCHMERZ. Pain associated with ovulation. It occurs usually at the time of ovulation, about halfway through the cycle. Translated, it means 'middle pain'.

NUTRITION. The British Society for Nutritional Medicine's definition is 'the sum of the processes involved in taking nutrients, assimilating and utilizing them'. In other words, the quality of the diet and the ability of your body to utilize the individual nutrients and so maintain health.

OESTROGEN. A steroid hormone which is produced in large quantities by the ovaries, and in smaller amounts by the adrenal glands. It is responsible for the development of breasts and other sexual characteristics at puberty. Oestrogen is also responsible for the production of fertile cervical mucus, the opening of the cervix, and building up of blood in the lining of the uterus, preparing for a fertilized egg.

OVARIES. A pair of glands situated on either side of the uterus, in which eggs and sex hormones, including oestrogen, are produced.

OVULATION. The release of the ripe egg (ovum) from the ovary. The two ovaries ovulate alternately every month. Occasionally, the two ovaries ovulate simultaneously, in which case the result may be twins.

OVUM. The egg which is released from the ovary at the time of ovulation.

PALPITATIONS. The heart beating too fast and sometimes irregularly.

PITUITARY GLAND. A small gland situated at the base of the brain, which produces many hormones, among which are those which stimulate the ovary and the thyroid.

PRE-MENSTRUAL. A term used to describe the time before the arrival of a period.

PRE-MENSTRUAL SYNDROME. This is the name given to a collection of mental and physical symptoms which manifest themselves before the onset of a period.

PRE-MENSTRUAL TENSION. This was the name first given to the symptoms detected before a period in 1931 by Dr Frank. Now the correct name is Pre-Menstrual Syndrome. However, many women still prefer to call the condition PMT – Pre-Menstrual Tension.

PROGESTERONE. A hormone secreted by the corpus luteum of the ovary during the second half of the menstrual cycle. Some studies have shown that a deficiency in progesterone may be responsible for some PMS symptoms. Progesterone is an important hormone during pregnancy.

PROGESTOGENS. A group of synthetic hormones, with actions similar to progesterone.

PROLACTIN. The hormone secreted by the pituitary gland which is involved in milk production. It is also known to affect water and mineral balance in the body, and in some women may play a part in the changes pre-menstrually.

PROSTAGLANDINS. Hormone-like substances found in almost every cell in the body, which are necessary for the normal function of involuntary muscles, including the heart, the uterus, blood vessels, the lungs and the intestines.

Prostaglandins are sometimes regarded as health controllers, as they seem to play an important part in the controlling of many essential functions in the body. They do not come directly from the diet, but are made in the body itself. Because of this, the body relies on a good diet in order to produce prostaglandins. The special substances that the body needs to make these hormones are called essential fatty acids.

SEROTONIN. A brain chemical that influences mood.

STEROIDS. Substances which have a particular chemical structure in common. All the sex hormones, such as oestrogen, progesterone, etc are steroids.

THYROID GLAND. A gland situated in the neck, which produces the hormone thyroxine. The thyroid gland regulates metabolism.

TRANQUILLIZERS. A group of drugs which artificially sedate the body. They may be useful in the short term, but in the long term they can have addictive qualities.

UTERUS (WOMB). A sac-like organ which is located in the abdomen of a woman, and designed to hold and nourish a growing child from conception until birth.

VAGINA. The passage that leads from the uterus to the external genital organs.

2 FOOD ADDITIVES

There are many types of food additives. Most of them are denoted by a number prefixed by E. The E stands for EEC, as the European Community Regulations state that, since 1 January 1986, all foods containing additives, except for flavourings, must have an E number, or the actual name, in the list of ingredients. Some food additives are natural, vegetable-derived compounds, or even vitamins, and are perfectly harmless. However, these are not used frequently. The following additives can be associated with the exacerbation of certain medical problems:

Azo-dyes E102, E104, E107, E110, E122, E123, E124, E128, E131, E132, E133, E142, E151, E154, E155, E180
Benzoates E210–E219
Sulphur dioxide and sulphites E220–E227
Nitrites and nitrates E249–E252
Proprionic acid and propionates E280–E283
Anti-oxidants, BHA & BHT E320 and E321
Monosodium glutamate (MSG) and related compounds E621–E623

Many food allergy associations now give details of suppliers of foods suitable for people who suffer from allergies. Some of these are mentioned on page 253. Many supermarkets will now provide lists of their products which are free from additives, milk, wheat, eggs, etc. For those who wish to request further details, it is suggested that you contact the customer relations department of the appropriate supermarket chain.

The Ministry of Agriculture, Fisheries and Food has produced a booklet explaining what the 'E' numbers mean. There is also the excellent book 'E for Additives' by Maurice Hanssen, which is readily available. An organization called 'Foresight', The Association for the Promotion of Pre-Conceptual Care, have produced a handbag-sized booklet based on the information from the book 'E for Additives'. They have marked additive numbers with a colour code, red for danger, and they specify precisely why, orange for those additives on which conflicting reports still exist, and green for those about which there are no known side-effects. This booklet is immensely valuable as it takes the confusion out of shopping. You will find the Foresight address in Appendix 5 should you wish to obtain a copy.

3 NUTRITIONAL SUPPLEMENT SUPPLIERS

1. Efamol — Boots, chemists, healthfood shops and Nutritional Health (mail order)*
2. Femvite — Nutritional Health (mail order)*. Available from chemists and healthfood shops in late 1994.
3. Linusit Gold — Healthfood shops.
4. Magnesium Hydroxide Mixture — Boots and other chemists.
5. Optivite — Boots, chemists, healthfood shops and Nutritional Health (mail order)*
6. Natural Vitamin E — Healthfood shops and Nutritional Health (mail order)*
7. Sugar Factor/Normoglycaemia — Nutritional Health (mail order)*

*Mail Order Address
Nutritional Health Ltd
PO Box 926
Lewes, East Sussex
BN7 2QL

Australia

NNFA (National Nutrition Foods Association)
PO Box 84, Westmead, NSW 2145. Tel: 02 633 9913
The NNFA have lists of all supplement stockists and retailers in Australia, if you have any difficulties in obtaining supplements.

New Zealand

NNFA (National Nutrition Foods Association)
c/o PO Box 820062, Auckland, New Zealand.
Again the NNFA have lists of all supplement stockists and retailers in New Zealand, if you have any difficulties in obtaining supplements.

4 RECOMMENDED READING LIST

NOTE
UK, USA and A denotes the following books are available in Great Britain, United States and Australia.

GENERAL HEALTH

1. *Pure, White and Deadly* by Professor John Yudkin (a book about sugar) price £9.95 (published by Viking).   **UK   A**
2. *Coming off Tranquillizers* by Dr Susan Trickett, price £1.99 (published by Thorsons).   **UK   USA   A** (Lothian Publishing Co).
3. *The Migraine Revolution – The New Drug-free Solution* by Dr John Mansfield, price £4.99 (published by Thorsons).   **UK   USA   A** (Lothian Publishing Co).
4. *Understanding Cystitis* by Angela Kilmartin, price £4.99 (published by Arrow Books).   **UK   A**
5. *The Book of Massage*, price £9.99 (published by Ebury Press).   **UK**
6. *Do-it-yourself Shiatsu* by W. Ohashi, price £5.50 (published by Unwin).   **UK**
7. *Candida Albicans: Could Yeast Be Your Problem?* by Leon Chaitow, price £3.99 (published by Thorsons).   **UK   USA   A** (Lothian Publishing Co).
8. *Candida Albicans* by Gill Jacobs, price £6.99 (published by Optima).   **UK   USA   A**
9. *Nutritional Medicine* by Dr Stephen Davies and Dr Alan Stewart, price £7.99 (published by Pan Books).   **UK   A**
10. *The Y Plan Countdown*, price £6.99 (published by Hamlyn).   **UK**
11. *Bone Boosters – Natural Ways to Beat Osteoporosis* by Diana Moran and Helen Franks, price £9.99 (published by Boxtree Limited).   **UK**
12. *The Migraine Handbook* by Jenny Lewis, price £6.99 (published by Vermilion).   **UK   A**
13. *The Book of Yoga*, Sivananda Yoga Centre, price £9.99 (published by Ebury Press).   **UK   A**

DIET

1. *The Vitality Diet* by Maryon Stewart and Dr Alan Stewart, price £4.99 (published by Optima).   **UK   A**
2. *Good Food Gluten-Free* by Hilda Cherry Hills, price £9.99 (published by Keats).   **USA**
3. *The Wheat and Gluten Free Cookbook* by Joan Noble, price £8.99 (published by Vermilion). **UK A**
4. *The New Why You Don't Need Meat* by Peter Cox, price £10.99 (published by Bloomsbury).   **UK   A**
5. *Beat Sugar Craving* by Maryon Stewart, price £7.99 (published by Vermilion).   **UK   A**
6. *The Allergy Diet* by Elizabeth Workman SRD, Dr John Hunter and Dr Virginia Alun Jones, price £3.99 (published by Martin Dunitz). **UK USA**
7. *The Candida Albicans Yeast-Free Cook Book* by Pat Connolly and Associates of the Price Pottenger Nutrition Foundation, price £6.95 (published by Keats Publishing Inc). **UK USA**

8. *The Cranks Recipe Book* by David Canter, Hay Canter and Daphne Swann, price £1.85 (published by Grafton). **UK**

9. *The Food Intolerance Diet* by Elizabeth Workman SRD, Dr Virginia Alun Jones and Dr John Hunter, price £3.95 (published by Martin Dunitz). **UK USA**

10. *Raw Energy* by Leslie and Susannah Kenton, price £6.99 (published by Vermilion). **UK A** (Doubleday Publishing Co).

11. *The Reluctant Vegetarian* by Simon Hope, price £8.95 (published by William Heinemann). **UK**

12. *The Salt-Free Diet Book* by Dr Graham McGregor, price £3.95 (published by Martin Dunitz). **UK USA**

13. *Gourmet Vegetarian Cooking* by Rose Elliot price £2.95 (published by Fontana). **UK A**

14. *Healthy Cooking,* price 0.99 from Tesco Stores. **UK**

15. *Food Allergy and Intolerance* by Jonathan Brostoff and Linda Gamlin, price £4.99 (published by Bloomsbury). **UK A**

16. *The Gluten-free and Wheat-free Bumper Bake Book* by Rita Greer, price £2.95 (published by Bunterbird Ltd). **UK**

STRESS

1. *Self-Help for your Nerves* by Dr Clair Weekes, price £5.95 (published by Angus and Robertson). **UK USA** (Hawthorn Publishing Co).

2. *Stress and Relaxation Self-Help Techniques for Everyone* by Jane Madders, price £6.99 (published by Optima). **UK USA A**

3. *Lyn Marshall's Instant Stress Cure,* price £8.99 (published by Vermilion). **UK A**

GENERAL

1. *How to Stop Smoking and Stay Stopped for Good* by Gillian Riley, price £5.99 (published by Vermilion). **UK A**

2. *Getting Sober and Loving It* by Joan and Derek Taylor, price £7.99 (published by Vermilion). **UK A**

3. *The National Childbirth Book of Breast Feeding* by Mary Smale, price £7.99 (published by Vermilion). **UK**

4. *Tired all the Time* by Dr Alan Stewart, price £6.99 (published by Optima). **UK USA A**

5. *Memory Power* by Ursula Markham, price £7.99 (published by Vermilion). **UK A**

6. *Alternative Health Aromatherapy* by Gill Martin, price £5.99 (published by Optima). **UK USA A**

7. *Alternative Health Acupuncture* by Dr Michael Nightingale, price £5.00 (published by Optima). **UK USA A**

8. *Alternative Health Osteopathy* by Stephen Sandler, price £5.99 (published by Optima). **UK USA A**

5 USEFUL ADDRESSES

GREAT BRITAIN

British Acupuncture Register and Directory
34 Alderney Street, London SW1V 4UE.   Tel: London (071) 834 1012.

The Council for Acupuncture
Suite 1, 19a Cavendish Square, London W1M 9AD.   Tel: London (071) 409 1440.

Alcoholics Anonymous (AA)
General Services Office, PO Box 1, Stonebow House, Stonebow, York YO1 2NJ.
Tel: York (0904) 644026.

Action Against Allergy
23–24 George Street, Richmond, Surrey TW9 1JY.

National Society for Research into Allergy
PO Box 45, Hinkley, Leicestershire LE10 1JY.   Tel: 0455 851546.

Anorexia and Bulimia Nervosa Association
Tottenham Women's and Health Centre, Annexe C, Tottenham Town Hall, Town Hall
Approach, London N15 4RX.   Tel: London (081) 885 3936 (Wednesdays
6–8.30 pm only)

International Federation of Aromatherapists
4 Eastmearn Road, West Dulwich, London SE21 8HA.
Letters only enclosing a sae.

British Pregnancy Advisory Service
7 Belgrave Road, London SW1V 1QB.   Tel: London (071) 222 0985.

Brook Advisory Centre
Head Office, 153a East Street, Walworth, London SE17 2SD.   Tel: London
(081) 708 1234.

CLEAR (Campaign for Lead Free Air)
3 Endsleigh Street, London WC1H 0DD.   Tel: London (071) 278 9686.

Hyperactive Children Support Group
59 Meadowside, Angmering, Littlehampton, West Sussex BN16 4BW.
(Postal enquiries only.)

ASSET
The National Association for Health and Exercise Teachers
202 The Avenue, Kennington, Oxford OX1 5RN.   Tel: Oxford (0865) 736066.

The Sports Council
16 Upper Woburn Place, London WC1H 0QP.   Tel: London (071) 388 1277.

Medau Society
8b Robson House, East Street, Epsom, Surrey KT17 1HH.   Tel: Epsom
(03727) 29056.

Endometriosis Society
35 Belgrave Square, London SW1X 8QB.   Tel: London (071) 235 4137.

Food Watch International
Butts Pond Industrial Estate, Sturminster Newton, Dorset DT10 1AZ.
Tel: Sturminster Newton (0258) 73356.

Foresight
Association for the Promotion of Pre-Conceptual Care
The Old Vicarage, Church Lane, Whitney, Godalming, Surrey GU8 5PN.
Tel: Wormley (042879) 4500.

Friends of the Earth Ltd
26–28 Underwood Street, London N1 7JQ.   Tel: London
(071 490 1555.

Migraine Trust
45 Great Ormond Street, London WC1 3HD.   Tel: London (071) 278 2676.

National Childbirth Trust
Alexander House, Oldham, London W3 6NH.   Tel: London (081) 992 8637.

The European School of Osteopathy
104 Tonbridge Road, Maidstone, Kent ME16 8SL.   Tel: Maidstone (0622) 671558.

The British School of Osteopathy
Little John House, 1–4 Suffolk Street, London SW1 4HG.   Tel: London
(071) 930 9254.

Patients Association
18 Victoria Park Square, Bethnal Green, London E2 9PF.   Tel: London
(071) 981 5676.

Action on Phobias
c/o Shandy Mathias, 8–9 The Avenue, Eastbourne, East Sussex BN21 2YA.
Letters only enclosing a sae.

The Women's Nutritional Advisory Service
PO Box 268, Lewes, East Sussex BN7 2QN.   Tel: Brighton (0273) 487366.

Association for Post-Natal Illness
7 Gowan Avenue, London SW6 6RH.   Tel: London (071) 731 4867.

Release
388 Old Street, London EC1V 9LT.   Tel: London (071) 729 9904.

Samaritans
10 The Grove, Slough SL1 1QP.   Tel: Slough (0753) 532713.

The Shiatsu Society
Elaine Liechti, 19 Langside Park, Kilbarchan, Renfrewshire PA10 2EP.
Tel: Kilbarchan (050 57) 4657.

The Henry Doubleday Research Association
Ryton Gardens, National Centre for organic gardening, Ryton on Dunsmore, Coventry
CV8 3LG.   Tel: Coventry (0203) 303517.

The Soil Association
86–88 Colston Street, Bristol BS1 5BB.   Tel: Bristol (0272) 290661.

Both these organizations advise on all aspects of non-chemical agriculture, give advice to
amateur and professional organic growers, and have a constantly updated list of sources of
organic produce.

Ash (Action on Smoking and Health)
5–11 Mortimer Street, London W1N 7RH.   Tel: London (071) 637 9843.

Tranx (UK) Ltd
National Tranquilliser Advice Centre, Registered Office, 25a Masons Avenue,
Wealdstone, Harrow, Middx HA3 5AH.   Tel: (client line) (081) 427 2065 [24-hour
answering service] (081) 427 2827.

AUSTRALIA

Blackmores Limited
23 Roseberry Street, Balgowlah, NSW 2093.   Tel: (02) 949 3177.

Royal Society for the Welfare of Mothers and Babies
2 Shaw Street, Petersham, NSW 2049.   Tel: (02) 568 3633.

Childbirth Education Association of Victoria
21 Greensborough Centre, 25 Main Street, Greensborough, Victoria 3088.

Women's Health Advisory Service
187 Glenmore Road, Paddington NSW 2021.   Tel: (02) 331 5014.

Liverpool Women's Health Centre
26 Bathurst Street, Liverpool NSW 2170.   Tel: (02) 601 3555.

Adelaide Women's Community Health
64 Pennington Terrace, Nth Adelaide SA 5006.   Tel: (08) 267 5366.

PMT Relief Clinic
Suite 6, 32 Kensington Road, Rose Park, South Australia 5067.   Tel: (08) 364 2760.

NEW ZEALAND

Papakura Women's Centre
4 Opaneke Road, Papakura, Auckland.   Tel: 299 9466.

Whakatane Women's Collective
PO Box 3049, Ohope.   Tel: (Whakatane) 076 24757.

Health Alternative for Women
Room 101, Cranmer Centre, PO Box 884, Christchurch.   Tel: 796 970.

Women's Health Collective
63 Ponsonby Road, Ponsonby, Auckland.   Tel: 764 506.

West Auckland Women's Centre
111 McLeod Road, Te Atatu, Auckland.   Tel: 8366 381.

Tauranga Women's Centre
PO Box 368, Tauranga.   Tel: 783 530.

The Alice Bush Family Planning Clinic
214 Karangahape Road, Auckland.   Tel: 775 049.

Family Planning Clinic
Arts Centre, 301 Montreal Street, Christchurch.   Tel: 790 514.

USA AND CANADA

National Institute of Nutrition
1565 Carling Avenue, #400, Ottawa, Ontario K12 8R1.

The American Academy of Environmental Medicine
PO Box 16106, Denver, Colorado, 80216.

Optimox Inc
PO Box 3378, Torrance, California 90510–3378.   Tel: (800) 223 1601.

6 CHARTS
AND DIARIES

SYMPTOMS	WEEK AFTER PERIOD (Fill in 3 days after period)				WEEK BEFORE PERIOD (Fill in 2-3 days before period)			
	None	Mild	Moderate	Severe	None	Mild	Moderate	Severe
PMS – A								
Nervous Tension								
Mood Swings								
Irritability								
Anxiety								
PMS - H								
Weight Gain								
Swelling of Extremities								
Breast Tenderness								
Abdominal Bloating								
PMS - C								
Headache								
Craving for Sweets								
Increased Appetite								
Heart Pounding								
Fatigue								
Dizziness or Fainting								
PMS - D								
Depression								
Forgetfulness								
Crying								
Confusion								
Insomnia								
OTHER SYMPTOMS								
Loss of Sexual Interest								
Disorientation								
Clumsiness								
Tremors/Shakes								
Thoughts of Suicide								
Agoraphobia								
Increased Physical Activity								
Heavy/Aching Legs								
Generalized Aches								
Bad Breath								
Sensitivity to Music/Light								
Excessive Thirst								

Do you have any other PRE-MENSTRUAL SYMPTOMS not listed opposite? Use this page to make a note of these. 'Weight Gain' in the chart opposite refers to the amount you put on before your period.

MENSTRUAL SYMPTOMATOLOGY DIARY

Month:_____

GRADING OF MENSES

0–none	3–heavy
1–slight	4–heavy and
2–moderate	clots

GRADING OF SYMPTOMS (COMPLAINTS)

0–none
1–mild-present but does not interfere with activities
2–moderate-present and interferes with activities but not disabling
3–severe-disabling. Unable to function.

Day of cycle																													
Date																													
Period																													

PMS - A

Nervous tension																													
Mood swings																													
Irritability																													
Anxiety																													

PMS - H

Weight gain																													
Swelling of extemities																													
Breast tenderness																													
Abdominal bloating																													

PMS - C

Headache																													
Craving for sweets																													
Increased appetite																													
Heart pounding																													
Fatigue																													
Dizziness or faintness																													

PMS - D

Depression																													
Forgetfulness																													
Crying																													
Confusion																													
Insomnia																													

PAIN

Cramps (low abdominal)																													
Backache																													
General aches/pains																													

NOTES:

MENSTRUAL SYMPTOMATOLOGY DIARY

Month: _____

GRADING OF MENSES

0–none	3–heavy
1–slight	4–heavy and
2–moderate	clots

GRADING OF SYMPTOMS (COMPLAINTS)

0–none
1–mild-present but does not interfere with activities
2–moderate-present and interferes with activities but not disabling
3–severe-disabling. Unable to function.

Day of cycle																													
Date																													
Period																													

PMS - A

Nervous tension																													
Mood swings																													
Irritability																													
Anxiety																													

PMS - H

Weight gain																													
Swelling of extemities																													
Breast tenderness																													
Abdominal bloating																													

PMS - C

Headache																													
Craving for sweets																													
Increased appetite																													
Heart pounding																													
Fatigue																													
Dizziness or faintness																													

PMS - D

Depression																													
Forgetfulness																													
Crying																													
Confusion																													
Insomnia																													

PAIN

Cramps (low abdominal)																													
Backache																													
General aches/pains																													

NOTES:

7 REFERENCES

Below is a list of some of the more important references relating to studies detailed in this edition of the book. The WNAS has endeavoured over the years to keep details of most of the important studies on the causation and treatment of PMS. A copy of these references and other information on PMS can be obtained from the WNAS by sending £3 in postage stamps to The Women's Nutritional Advisory Service, PO Box 268, Lewes, Sussex BN7 2QN.

Chapter 1

1. Green R., Dalton K. The Pre-Menstrual Syndrome. British Medical Journal. May 9, 1953. P1007–1014.
2. Abraham G.E. Nutrition and the Pre-Menstrual Tension Syndromes. Journal of Applied Nutrition. 36:103–124. 1984.
3. Morton J.H., Additon H., Addison R.G., Hunt L., Sullivan J.J. A clinical study of Pre-Menstrual Tension. A.M.J.Obstet.Gynecol. 55:1182–1191. 1953.

Chapter 2

1. Abraham G.E. Management of the Pre-Menstrual Tension Syndromes: Rationale for a Nutritional Approach. In: A Year in Nutritional Medicine, Second Edition 1986. Ed. by Bland J. Keats Publishing, Inc. New Canaan, Connecticut: 125–166. 1986.
2. Munday M.R., Brush M.G., Taylor R.W. Correlation between Progesterone, Oestradiol and Aldosterone Levels in the Pre-Menstrual Syndrome. Clinical Endocrinology. 14:1–9. 1981.
3. Watts J.F.F., Butt W.P., Logan Edwards R., Holder G. Hormonal Studies in Women with Pre-Menstrual Tension. British Journal of Obstetrics and Gynaecology. 92:247–255. 1985.
4. Dalton M.E. Sex Hormone-Binding Globulin Concentrations in Women with Severe Pre-Menstrual Syndrome. Post-Graduate Medical Journal. 57:560–561. 1981.

Chapter 3

1. Moos R.H. Typology of Menstrual Cycle Symptoms. American Journal of Obstet.Gynec. 103:390–402. 1969.

Chapter 4

1. Dalton K. Pre-Menstrual Syndrome and Progesterone Therapy. Second Edition. William Heinemann Medical Books Limited London. 1984.
2. Hargrove J.T., Abraham G.E. The Incidence of Pre-Menstrual Tension in a Gynaecologic Clinic. The Journal of Reproductive Medicine. 27:721–724. 1982.
3. Hargrove J.T., Abraham G.E. The Ubiquitousness of Pre-Menstrual Tension in a Gynaecologic Practice. The Journal of Reproductive Medicine. 28:435–437. 1983.

Chapter 5

1. Yudkin J. Pure, White and Deadly. Viking Press. London. 1986.
2. Royal College of General Practitioners. Alcohol – A Balanced View. Report from General Practice 24. RCGP London. 1986.
3. Drug Abuse Briefing. Institute for the Study of Drug Dependents. London. 1986.
4. Abraham G.E. Nutrition and the Pre-Menstrual Tension Syndromes. Journal of Applied Nutrition. 36:103–124. 1984.

5. Ashton C.H. Caffeine and Health. The British Medical Journal. 295:1293–4. 1987.

Chapter 6

1. Boyle C.A. et al. Caffeine Consumption and Fibrocystic Breast Disease: A Case-Control Epidemiologic Study. JNCI. 72:1015–1019. 1984.
2. O'Brien P.M.S, Selby C., Symonds E.N. Progesterone, Fluid and Electrolytes in Pre-Menstrual Syndrome. The British Medical Journal. 10 May 1980: 1161–1163.
3. MacGregor G.A. et al. Is 'Idiopathic' Oedema Idiopathic. The Lancet 1:397–400. 1979.
4. O'Brien P.M.S., Selby C., Symonds E.M. Progesterone, Fluid and Electrolytes in Pre-Menstrual Syndrome. The British Medical Journal. 280:1161–3. 1980.

Chapter 7

1. Yudkin J. Pure, White and Deadly. Viking Press. London. 1986.
2. Morton J.H., Additon H., Addison R.G., Hunt L., Sullivan J.J. A clinical study of Pre-Menstrual Tension. A.M.J.Obstet.Gynecol. 55:1182–1191. 1953.

Chapter 8

1. Abraham G.E. Nutrition and the Pre-Menstrual Tension Syndromes. Journal of Applied Nutrition. 36:103-124. 1984.
2. Dalton K. Pre-Menstrual Syndrome and Progesterone Therapy. Second Edition. William Heinemann Medical Books Limited London. 1984.

Chapter 9

1. Dalton K. Pre-Menstrual Syndrome and Progesterone Therapy. Second Edition. William Heinemann Medical Books Limited London. 1984.

Chapter 10

1. Pre-Menstrual Syndrome – Proceedings for Workshop held at the Royal College of Obstetricians and Gynaecologists. London, 2nd December 1982. Ed. Taylor. R.W. Medical News – Tribune Limited. London. 1983.
2. Sampson J.A. Pre-Menstrual Syndrome: A Double-Blind Control Trial of Progesterone and Placebo. British Journal of Psychiatry. 135:209–215. 1979.
3. Dennerstein L., et al. Progesterone and the Pre-Menstrual Syndrome: A Double-Blind Cross Over Trial. British Medical Journal. 290:1617–1621. 1985.
4. Magos A., Studd J. Progesterone and the Pre-Menstrual Syndrome: A Double-Blind Cross Over Trial. British Medical Journal. 291:213–214. 1985.
5. O'Brien P.M.S. The Pre-Menstrual Syndrome: A Review of the Present Status of Therapy. Drugs 24:140–151. 1982.

Chapter 11

1. Modern Nutrition in Health and Disease. Ed: Goodhart R.S., Shils M.E. Sixth edition Lea and Febiter, Philadelphia. 1980.
2. Nutritional Medicine. Davies S., Stewart A. Pan Books London. 1987.
3. Lewis J., Buss D.H. Trace Nutrients 5. Minerals and Vitamins in the British Household Food Supply. British Journal of Nutrition. 60:413–424. 1988.
4. Spring J.A., Robertson J., Buss D.H. British Journal of Nutrition. 41:487–493. 1979.
5. Gregory J., Foster K., Tyler H. and Wiseman M. The Dietary and Nutritional Survey of British Adults. HMSO. London 1990.
6. Committee on Medical Aspects of Food Policy. Dietary Reference Values for Food Energy and Nutrients for the United Kingdom. HMSO. London 1991.

Chapter 12

1. Piesse. J.W. Nutrition Factors in the Pre-Menstrual Syndrome. International Clinical Nutrition Review. 4:54–81. 1984.
2. Hargrove J.T., Abraham G.E. Effect of Vitamin B6 on Infertility in Women with Pre-Menstrual Syndrome. Infertility 2:315–322. 1979.
3. Abraham G.E., Hargrove J.T. The Effect of Vitamin B6 on Pre-Menstrual Symptomatology in Women with Pre-Menstrual Syndrome: A Double-Blind Cross Over Study. Infertility. 3:155–165. 1980.
4. Gunn A.D.G. Vitamin B6 and the Pre-Menstrual Syndrome. In Vitamins-Nutrients as Therapeutic Agents. Ed: Hanck A., Hornig D. Hans Huber Publishers. Bern. 1985. P213–224.
5. Stokes J., Mendels J. Pyridoxine and Pre-Menstrual Tension. The Lancet 1:1177–1178. 1972.
6. Abraham G.E. Magnesium Deficiency in Pre-Menstrual Tension. Magnesium Bulletin 1:68–73. 1982.
7. Abraham G.E., Lubran M.M. Serum and Red Cell Magnesium levels in patients with Pre-Menstrual Tension. The American Journal of Clinical Nutrition. 34:2364–2366. 1981.
8. Sherwood R.A., Rocks B.F., Stewart A., Saxton R.S. Magnesium in the Pre-Menstrual Syndrome. Ann. Clin. Biochem. 23:667–670. 1986.
9. Pre-Menstrual Tension: An Invitation a Symposium. Ed. Abraham G.E. Journal of Reproductive Medicine. 28:7 & 8:433–538. 1983.
10. Fushs N., Hakim M., Abraham G.E. The Effect of a Nutritional Supplement, Optivite, for Women with Pre-Menstrual Tension Syndromes. 1. Effect of Blood Chemistry and Serum Steroid levels during the mid-luteal phase. The Journal of Applied Nutrition. 37:1–11. 1986.
11. Chakmakjian Z.H., Higgins C.E., Abraham G.E. The Effect of a Nutritional Supplement, Optivite, for Women, on Pre-Menstrual Tension Syndromes: 2. The effect of Symptomatology, using a Double-Blind Cross-Over Design. The Journal of Applied Nutrition. 37:12–17. 1986.
12. London, R.S. et al. The Effect of Alpha-Tocopherol on Pre-Menstrual Symptomatology: A Double-Blind Study. Journal of the American College of Nutrition. 2:115–122. 1983.
13. London, R.S. et al. The Effect of Alpha-Tocopherol on Pre-Menstrual Symptomatology: A Double-Blind Study 2. Endocrine correlates. Journal of the American College of Nutrition. 3:351–356. 1984.
14. O'Brien P.M.S. Pre-Menstrual Syndrome. Blackwell Scientific Publications, Oxford, 1987.
15. Stewart A.A. Rational Approach to Treating Pre-Menstrual Syndrome. WNAS publication, 1989.
16. Stewart A. Clinical and Biochemical Effects of Nutritional Supplementation on the Pre-Menstrual Syndrome. The Journal of Reproductive Medicine. 32:435–441. 1987.
17. Boyd E.M.F. et al. The effect of a low-fat, high complex-carbohydrate diet on symptoms of cyclical mastopathy. The Lancet. 2:128–132. 1988.
18. Freeman E., Rickels K., Sondheimer S.J. and Polansky M. Ineffectiveness of Progesterone Suppository Treatment for Pre-Menstrual Syndrome. Journal of the American Medical Association. 264:349–53. 1990.
19. Kleijnen J., ter Riet G. and Knipschild P. Vitamin B6 in the Treatment of Pre-Menstrual Syndrome: A Review. British Journal of Obstetrics and Gynaecology. 97:847–852. 1990.
20. London R.S., Bradley L. and Chiamori N.Y. Effect of a Nutritional Supplement on Pre-Menstrual Symptomatology in Women with Pre-Menstrual Syndrome: A Double-Blind Longitudinal Study. Journal of the American College of Nutrition. 10:494–499. 1991.

Chapter 14

1. Yudkin J. Pure, White and Deadly. Viking Press, London. 1986.
2. Royal College of General Practitioners. Alcohol – A Balanced View. Report from General Practice, 24. RCGP. London 1986.
3. Health Education Council. That's The Limit – Booklet. HEC, 78 New Oxford Street, London EC1A 1AH.
4. Nutritional Medicine by Dr Stephen Davies and Dr Alan Stewart. Pan Books. 1987.
5. Which? Troubled Waters, Which? November 1986. P494–497.
6. Spring J.A., Robertson J., Buss D.H. Trace Nutrients 3. Magnesium, Copper, Zinc, Vitamin B6, Vitamin B12 and Folic Acid in the British Household Food Supply. Br.J.Nutr. 41:487–493. 1979.
7. Victor B.S., Greden J.F., and Lubetsky, M. Somatic Manifestations of Caffeinism. J.Clin Psychiat. 42:185–8. 1981.
8. Disler P.B. et al. The Effects of Tea on Iron Absorption. Gut 18:193–200. 1975.
9. Tonkin S.Y. Vitamins and Oral Contraceptives. In Vitamins in Human Biology in Medicine. Ed: Briggs M.H. CRC Press, Boca Raton, Florida. P29–64. 1981.
10. Walters A.H., Fletcher, J.R., Law S.J. Nitrate in Vegetables: Estimation by HPLC. Nutrition and Health. 4:141–149. 1986.
11. Mount J.L. The Food and Health of Western Man. Charles Knight & Co Ltd, London. 1975.
12. The Booker Health Report – A Survey of Vitamin and Mineral Intakes within Certain Population Groups. Booker Health Foods. 1986.

Chapter 19

1. Chuong C.J., Coulam C.B., Kao P.C., Bergstalh J., Go V.L.W. Neuropeptide levels in Pre-Menstrual Syndrome. Fertility and Sterility. 44:760–765. 1985.
2. Prior J.C., Vigna Y. and Alojada N. Conditioning Exercise Decreases Pre-Menstrual Symptoms. European Journal of Applied Physiology. 55:349–355. 1986.

INDEX

FURTHER HELP

If you would like information on the WNAS programme for pre-menstrual syndrome, or want to let me know about your success using the recommendations in this book, you can write to me at the following address.

If you require information, a large (A4) stamped, self-addressed envelope will guarantee you a reply; please state particularly that you are interested in receiving information on PMS, as we help women with all sorts of other conditions as well (see below).

Women's Nutritional Advisory Service
PO Box 268
Lewes
East Sussex BN7 2QN.

ADVICE LINES
FROM THE WNAS

OVERCOME PMS NATURALLY	0839 556600
THE PMS DIET LINE	0839 556601
OVERCOME MENOPAUSE NATURALLY	0839 556602
THE MENOPAUSE DIET LINE	0839 556603
BEAT SUGAR CRAVING	0839 556604
THE VITALITY DIET LINE	0839 556605
OVERCOMING BREAST TENDERNESS	0839 556606
OVERCOME PERIOD PAINS NATURALLY	0839 556607
GET FIT FOR PREGNANCY AND BREASTFEEDING	0839 556608
SKIN, NAIL & HAIR SIGNS OF DEFICIENCY	0839 556609
IMPROVE LIBIDO NATURALLY	0839 556610
BEAT IRRITABLE BOWEL SYNDROME	0839 556611
OVERCOME FATIGUE	0839 556612
BEAT MIGRAINE NATURALLY	0839 556613
OVERCOME OVULATION PAIN	0839 556614
DIRECTORY	0839 556615